NEITHER GODS NOR BEASTS

HOW SCIENCE IS CHANGING
WHO WE THINK WE ARE

Also From Cold Spring Harbor Laboratory Press

Abraham Lincoln's DNA and Other Adventures in Genetics

The Eighth Day of Creation: Makers of the Revolution in Biology

The Inside Story: DNA to RNA to Protein

I Wish I'd Made You Angry Earlier: Essays on Science, Scientists, and Humanity

Max Perutz and the Secret of Life

Phage and the Origins of Molecular Biology, The Centennial Edition

The Strongest Boy in the World: How Genetic Information Is Reshaping Our Lives

Other Titles by Elof Axel Carlson

Mendel's Legacy: The Origin of Classical Genetics

Times of Triumph, Times of Doubt: Science and the Battle for Public Trust

The Unfit: A History of a Bad Idea

NEITHER GODS NOR BEASTS

HOW SCIENCE IS CHANGING WHO WE THINK WE ARE

Elof Axel Carlson

COLD SPRING HARBOR LABORATORY PRESS
Cold Spring Harbor, New York • www.cshlpress.com

NEITHER GODS NOR BEASTS
How Science Is Changing Who We Think We Are

Publisher	John Inglis
Acquisition & Developmental Editor	Judy Cuddihy
Development, Marketing, & Sales Director	Jan Argentine
Project Coordinator	Mary Cozza
Production Editor	Kaaren Hegquist
Desktop Editor	Lauren Heller
Production Manager	Denise Weiss
Book Marketing Manager	Ingrid Benirschke
Sales Account Manager	Elizabeth Powers
Cover Designer	Ed Atkeson

Front cover artwork: Antony Gormley, ANOTHER PLACE, 1997. Cast iron. 100 elements/ 189 × 53 × 29 cm. Installation view, Stavanger, Norway, 1998. Photograph taken by Dag Mirestrand. © Courtesy of the artist & Jay Jopling/White Cube.

Library of Congress Cataloging-in-Publication Data

Carlson, Elof Axel.
  Neither gods nor beasts : how science is changing who we think we are /
Elof Axel Carlson.
    p. cm.
  Includes bibliographical references and index.
  ISBN 978-0-87969-786-0 (hard cover : alk. paper)
  1. Science–Social aspects. 2. Science and civilization. 3.
Science–Philosophy. I. Title. II. Series.

Q175.5.C37 2008
303.48'3–dc22   2008001261

10 9 8 7 6 5 4 3 2 1

All World Wide Web addresses are accurate to the best of our knowledge at the time of printing.

All Cold Spring Harbor Laboratory Press publications may be ordered directly from Cold Spring Harbor Laboratory Press, 500 Sunnyside Blvd., Woodbury, New York 11797-2924. Phone: 1-800-843-4388 in Continental U.S. and Canada. All other locations: (516) 422-4100. FAX: (516) 422-4097. E-mail: cshpress@cshl.edu. For a complete catalog of all Cold Spring Harbor Laboratory Press publications, visit our World Wide Web Site http://www.cshlpress.com/.

Dedicated to my graduate Ph.D. students
at UCLA, 1960–1968

John Southin
Ronald Sederoff
Harry Corwin
Robert Hendrickson
John Jenkins
Dale Grace

Contents

Preface

————

ALTHOUGH THIS IS THE BEGINNING of the third millennium in the calendar system we today call C.E., or the Common Era, most of humanity has an outmoded and inadequate perception of human life that is better suited for living in the first or second millennium. To live in the third millennium, we have to be knowledgeable about science in the way that we are knowledgeable about history, literature, or politics. I do not mean we have to become scientists or know knowledge at the level of sophistication of scientists. After all, we do not expect our students to be expert historians or literary critics if they have the passing knowledge of American history or the world literature considered essential in a college-level liberal arts education.

But, what is missing that our largely liberal arts education fails to provide is a knowledge of science germane to the human condition. Citizens and their legislators are not well-informed about the science involved in global warming, stem cell research, DNA science, evolution, industrial waste disposal, hazards to our health, the influence of population growth on resources we call natural, energy alternatives to fossil fuels, and many other issues that dominate our news.

The third millennium will be science-saturated. It will change the way we think of ourselves. The view of human nature or the human condition we have today is a continuation of a view that is flawed about who we are, how we came into being, how our bodies work, and how our brains produce our minds. What will remain unchanged is our need for values, ideals to live by, and the pleasures of art, music, literature, and other ways the humanities and fine arts permeate and enrich our beings.

Yet, these arts and humanities are insufficient to give us a complete understanding of the world that we need to inhabit during the third millennium.

In *Neither Gods Nor Beasts: How Science Is Changing Who We Think We Are*, I attempt to show what our present view of human nature is like, how it came into being, why it is inadequate, and how we can enrich that understanding through knowledge of science. This book is also a plea to rethink how we teach science to our citizens and to take it seriously from kindergarten through grade 12 and in the first four years of college. I am not advocating scientism as a replacement for our top-heavy emphasis on the arts and humanities. Nor am I advocating that faith-based beliefs are irrelevant or wrong for those whose needs demand them. What I am advocating is a closer relation of the world views of the liberal arts and the sciences, so we can have better-informed legislative representatives, better-informed citizens, and a shift in priorities to give us a view of our humanity that is healthier, safer, more enlightened, and more thrilling to contemplate.

The title reflects the changing perception of what it means to be human. Each generation slightly alters that interpretation. We are too diverse as a species, with many personalities, religions, and cultures. Finding a consensus that defines us is unlikely. We are clearly not gods, but we are sometimes accused of playing God. We are not beasts, although in our worst behavior we can act that way. Being human allows us to reflect on who we are. In the past, those reflections involved little scientific knowledge of the universe, living and inanimate. Today, we are engulfed in new knowledge that, I believe, is changing who we think we are.

I like to think that I am at home in the sciences and the humanities. I have read widely in both of these broad ways of interpreting human life, and this book is an effort to bring to those in the humanities some of the ways science alters our sense of who we are. It is also intended for my fellow scientists who may not appreciate as much as those in the humanities, the importance of considering the Golden Rule as a guide to the applications of science. The history of science is studded with bad outcomes because those using science have often ignored the empathy inherent in the Golden Rule. I doubt any of my readers wish to be killed, imprisoned, beaten, intimidated, robbed, or lied to all in the name of a higher cause, whether that is someone else's religious, national, ideological, or familial loyalty. I think that message is important and it is for that reason I have written this book.

This is a book that reflects a lifetime of reading and thinking about the role of science in our lives. For forty years, I taught a biology course for nonscience majors that attempted to inform students of the science they needed to know to engage in debates and make decisions for their health and their family. This is not a detailed history of how human nature and the human condition have changed over the millennia. For that reason, I did not use footnotes. Instead, I consider this a reasoned argument that readers may or may not accept, but which, I hope, will stimulate their thinking about who we are.

I thank Philip Reilly for his careful and thoughtful reading of this manuscript. Over the years, I have discussed what it means to be human with students and colleagues. I am particularly grateful to A. Peter Gary, Roderick Gorney, Paul Bingham, Paul Adams, Seymour Halperin, Howard Diamond, Mark Italiano, Owen Debowy, and Charles Spielholtz for their insights. I also thank Judy Cuddihy for her faith, encouragement, and skill in seeing this book evolve. The Cold Spring Harbor Laboratory Press staff have been dedicated and enthusiastic in working on this book. Thank you John Inglis, Denise Weiss, Mary Cozza, Kaaren Hegquist, Lauren Heller, and Jan Argentine. Finally, I thank my wife, Nedra, for her discussion and reading of the book from its germination as an idea to its fruition as a published work.

ELOF AXEL CARLSON
Setauket, New York

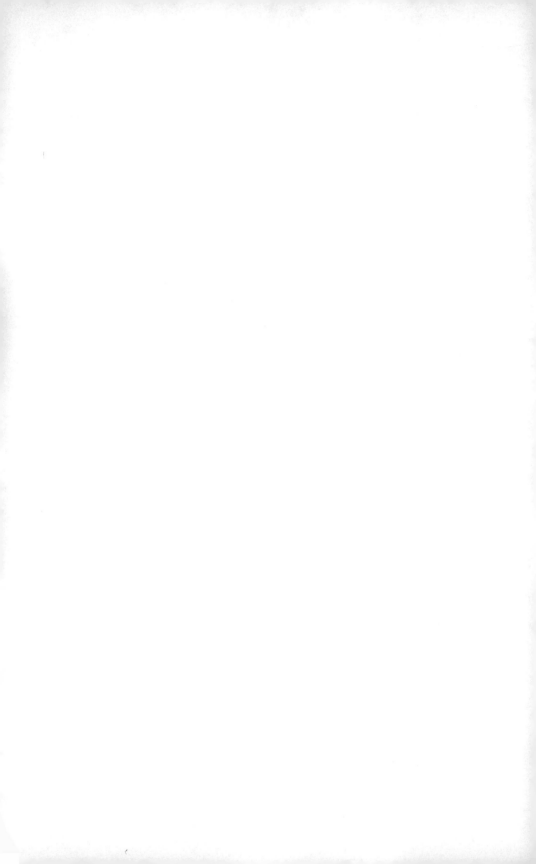

CHAPTER 1

Introduction

SCIENCE TODAY IS VERY DIFFERENT from the science of 100 years ago and even more different from that of 500 years ago. If you lived 500 years ago, you would not know that your body is composed of cells. You would not know that you transmit hereditary traits through genes, nor that infectious diseases are caused by small living things called microbes. You would soon know that your blood circulates and a bit later that capillaries connect the flow of blood between your arteries and veins. You would believe that all humans are descendants of Adam and Eve, who were created by God in his image. To your sixteenth-century self, science would be the way to read God's mind. You would believe that the largest object in the universe is the earth and that the sun, moon, planets, and stars all moved daily in circular orbits around the earth. You would believe that Kings are divinely ordained to rule you. You would consider slavery a natural status for those fated by their transgressions (or their ancestors' transgressions) to serve others. It would also seem natural to you that half of your children would die in their infancy.

As a person living in the twenty-first century, the scientific knowledge you do know (or benefit from) is on a much larger and smaller scale—from the immensity of the known universe to the infinitesimal interplay of subatomic particles. This knowledge has not changed your capacity to experience sorrow, accidents, the death of loved ones, happiness, love, fear, and uncertainty. In all likelihood, it never will. The range of human emotions is as true for those living 500 years ago as it is today. What has changed is your awareness that you can avoid a lot of harm that once seemed inevitable and that you have more control over your life than anyone in the 1500s thought possible. What has changed is not human nature (if we have one) but the human condition.

The Human Condition Is Not Human Nature

The human condition is descriptive and arises from our changing circumstances. Human nature, as most people imagine it, is claimed to be universal and innate. If we were to describe the human condition in 1500 in Europe, we would know that life for most of humanity was shorter and so were people—the mean life expectancy was about 35 years and the average adult height was about 2 inches less than it is today. Infant mortality caused most of the depression in life expectancy. The major causes of death were infectious diseases. We would take it for granted that there are the royalty, the clergy, and everyone else (the laity). If we were not royals or clergy, we would accept it as God's will that we were born to be peasants or born into a guild family so that we knew what our occupation would be by looking at our parents. Women, with few exceptions, were limited to being mothers or nuns. Most of humanity in 1500 in Europe was illiterate.

Most twenty-first-century North Americans and Europeans expect to live in a democracy. We are literate, with at least 12 years of schooling, and have many opportunities to work in a variety of occupations or professions. Women are equally schooled as men. Our life expectancy is close to 80 years of age. We can practice family planning to decide how many children we want and how to space them. We consider slavery a crime. We consider our success in life to be determined largely by talent and motivation and not by fate.

We had cultures and cities before we had formal occupations that we associate with science. We domesticated animals and plants before we knew how heredity works. We built bridges, temples, and canals before there were advanced mathematical skills, such as calculus, associated with engineering. In one sense, humans are no smarter today than they were 20,000 years ago. But knowledge is cumulative, and with the development of language, humans could store that knowledge and pass it on from parent to child, from guild member to guild apprentice, and from schoolteacher to schoolchild. In general, what worked and what was useful were preserved and what was false or harmful was rejected and forgotten or served as a cautionary tale.

What Does Make Us Human?

We distinguish ourselves from other animals by denying or minimizing our animality. One effective invention to do this was the belief that humans have a soul or spirit that other animals lacked or that differs in kind from the spirits that other animals possess. That special mental humanness allowed us to repudiate or discipline our animality (think of medieval practices such as mortification of the flesh). We were not gods and so we had to live with our bodily functions and urges. But because we considered ourselves special, we had to hide those functions from view and not dwell on them, at least not in public. I say this not to condemn our privacy but to understand why it is important to humans to separate our cultural lives from our animal lives that we encounter in the privacy of our bedrooms, bathrooms, and our passing thoughts.

In this book, I argue that it is important to know our animality, our biology, and our functions down to the molecular level. I show that such knowledge enriches us and does not lead to the fears of some critics of science who imagine such knowledge as diminishing human dignity, reducing humans to bestial behavior, or cauterizing our capacity for the good, the true, or the beautiful. I argue that what makes us human is our capacity to reason.

We learn poorly, if at all, from revelation, from intuition, from hearsay, or from superstition. What distinguishes the human mind from the minds of most animals is our capacity to use reason to figure out how the universe works, what our place in that universe is, and how we can provide a world more humane for our children than what we ourselves experienced. Does this mean we should live by reason alone? That is surely false because much of life is aesthetic and reflected in our arts. Much of our life involves making moral decisions about how we should respond to each other. It may be more rational to reject our family and to live with a far wealthier and better-educated family, but we rarely do this (even if that preferred family were willing to accept us) because we have values such as loyalty, kinship feelings, and emotional ties to our family, culture, religion, or nation. Yet, many people have made such choices by emigrating to America from other countries, leaving their relatives behind, learning a new language, and finding deep satisfaction in the newly acquired values of being American. Some changed their names, converted to other religions, and looked more with pity than admiration for their roots in "the old country." Their Americanized descendants, one or more generations later, may resurrect a nostalgic ethnic identity for those ancestral roots. If the history of families in America over several centuries is followed, most of those descendants will have mixed ethnic components and harbor no strong attachment to any of them.

Because all Americans are immigrants from other countries, including Native Americans who came from Asia in prehistoric times, we would not look upon the first ancestor in our line to come to these shores as having been less than human in rejecting the virtue of loyalty that bound that ancestor in another country. Something motivated that ancestor to seek a new life. It might have been opportunity, religious freedom, fear of persecution, loss of status in one's family, rejection of fighting in wars of questionable value, escaping debt, fear of criminal prosecution, or adventure. Humans are curiously motivated and it is the human condition, not human nature, that makes us pull up stakes and move on or stay put in an awkward situation. We are not likely to be born with genes for dogged loyalty or genes for itchy feet.

How Does Science Add to Our Humanity?

We learn about our place in the universe from four principal sources: revelation, tradition, experience, and science. Those who rely on revelation usually find that knowledge in religious texts. It is a knowledge based on faith. Why is it faith-based? The simplest answer comes from the plurality of religions and how religions change over time. The relation of humans to their universe differs among Jews, Catholics, Protestants, Moslems, Buddhists, Confucians, and hundreds of smaller religions. Some religions believe that people have souls and others do not. Some believe that there is a heaven and a hell and some do not. Some believe that they will retain their individuality after death forever and some believe that if they are lucky, they will merge with the godhead. Some believe that death is followed by nothingness. Some believe that their legacy is through their works or through their offspring. Some believe that their religion is right and all other religions are wrong. Some believe that there are many paths to wisdom, enlightenment, salvation, happiness, or satisfaction of living a life worth living. This tells us that revelation requires faith because all of these views cannot be simultaneously true, and none of them can be proven.

Tradition is passed on by culture. We mimic what our parents, neighbors, and other peers do. We may dress like them, share their musical tastes, develop a preference for our own foods, and have occupations often based on our family expectations. Traditions can be religious or secular. Our patriotism, our national holidays, and our class loyalties are filled with traditions passed from generation to generation. We rarely examine these traditions. They are based more on habit than on reason. With rare exceptions, we do not challenge them because most of them fit our needs and expectations. They are challenged when the human condition changes. It may have suited white people to have segregation as a way of life in the United States; however, it did not suit black people, and they led a civil rights revolution in the 1960s that changed tradition.

Experience is personal. Most children learn to avoid hurting themselves by actually hurting themselves or barely escaping harm. Idealism can be shattered by experience, as almost every black child growing up in the era before the civil rights revolution discovered. They had to know their place in a white supremacist world or face unhappy consequences. We often learn our limits through experience. Generations of college students learn how much their bodies can take staying awake and going to class with little sleep. They learn by experience how much alcohol abuse their bodies can take without leading to sickness or foolish behavior. Learning by experience is often effective, but it can be at considerable cost in damage to the body and to the ego. It is chiefly a secular way to learn.

Science is the exploration of the universe by reason, using standards of objectivity, controlled experimentation, verification of findings and interpretations by others, and recognition that theories that bind together a lot of facts may sometimes be wrong. In contrast to revelation, science demands evidence and keeps testing that evidence. Science gives us instruments to see the very small and the very large, and in so doing, it reveals worlds and levels of understanding that were not known to those experiencing revelations about the universe and our place in it several centuries or thousands of years ago. Galaxies, genes, chromosomes, cells, atoms, chemical molecules, weather forecasting, genetic counseling, antibiotics, nuclear energy, computers, and the medical treatment of sterility were largely unknown until the twentieth century. Science is mostly of recent origin in our world view. It often takes us by surprise and it sometimes contradicts the beliefs generated by those who derived their knowledge of the universe through revelation and the authority of scriptural texts.

Science often contradicts tradition and revelation. Its findings are universal, and what a scientist finds can be tested independently by scientists throughout the world. In fact, science requires its findings to be constantly tested and challenged. Knowledge by revelation does not. Revelation is inherently parochial because different religions have different revelations given to prophets. Revelation requires faith to believe in the legitimacy of the prophet's teachings. Science rejects using faith to justify its scientific findings. Reason, experimentation, observation, and the integrity of interpreting data with independent confirmation are essentials of science.

Science adds to our sense of who we are because we can now describe ourselves at anatomical, cellular, and molecular levels. We can follow our life cycle from fertilization through embryonic organ formation and from birth to death. We can now inventory our genes and use that knowledge to compare our genes, and the sequence of nucleotides for those genes, with those of other animals, plants, and microbes. It gives us more control over our destinies and diminishes fatalism. Science also forces us to think more deeply about values and applications of science to our bodies, to our environments, and to culture.

In this book, I introduce a brief overview of biology from a human perspective. We need to know that we are composed of cells, that genes specify all the components of our cells, that life operates at a molecular level, that we go through a life cycle, and that we evolve. We also need to know that what we call our mind is produced by the neurons of our brains and that neuronal activity is rapidly being interpreted at a molecular level. These ideas are not easy to assimilate for those whose knowledge of science is meager and so I have tried to minimize jargon and place concepts that are likely to be unfamiliar in a context that we can relate to as parents or citizens.

I argue that the fear of science and the rejection of scientific findings are hazardous to our health and to the future in which our descendants will live. We have profoundly altered the world we live in, largely by ignorance and selfishness. We will have to alter that world profoundly to restore what we take for granted, so that we will have a climate where we can live comfortably in the rhythm of our seasons with a minimum of floods, hurricanes, tornadoes, fires, and droughts. We want our descendants to live a life with sufficient food, healthy air and water, and a variety of landscapes to enjoy. If our shores are pushed inland by dozens or hundreds of miles as sea levels rise, we will have caused major disruptions in the lives of our descendants.

Science can predict bad outcomes from the careless habits of humanity. It can also be used to prevent such bad outcomes from happening. Being human means using our minds to distinguish these outcomes and to choose wisely. This cannot be done without knowledge of science. Muddling through may work in an era of ignorance, but it cannot work when science gives us powerful technologies that alter the world. This book is a plea for a more effective science education and a realization that the applications of science work best when those using it incorporate the idea of the Golden Rule into their thoughts and values.

Recommended Reading

Barbara Tuchman's *A distant mirror: The calamitous 14th century* (1996. Ballantine Books, New York) provides a view of what the human condition was like in the Middle Ages.

For a critique of learning by revelation, scriptural authority, or other supernatural sources, see Victor J. Stenger's *God: The failed hypothesis: How science shows that God does not exist* (2007. Prometheus Press, Amherst, New York). Also see Carl Sagan and Ann Druyan's *The demon haunted world: Science as a candle in the dark* (1997. Ballantine Books, New York).

For a view of science from a philosopher's perspective, I recommend Bertrand Russell's *The scientific outlook* (1931. W.W. Norton, New York).

PART 1

Humanity in a Prescientific Universe

S CIENCE IS A RELATIVELY NEW WAY of understanding the universe. Before the revolutionary findings of astronomy and anatomy in the sixteenth centuries, our knowledge of what is outside our bodies and what is inside our bodies was primitive, filled with errors, and left us dependent on faith-based knowledge or guesswork of who we were and what our place was in the universe. Humans do not need science to survive, but they do need reason to protect themselves, to learn from experience, and to be innovative. We know this because most of our time on earth as a species has been steeped in a world void of science.

If there is no science, how do we learn about the universe? To do this, we depended on supernatural explanations and concepts that assigned the existence of souls or spirits to humans and allowed us to create our religions. Many of these older ways of looking at ourselves and the world around us are gone in contemporary society. We have abandoned animism, a belief that everything that moves—from branches swaying in the wind to rocks tumbling down a cliff—is possessed by spirits of some sort. We have abandoned concepts that objects possess the Oceanic culture's concept of "mana," some vague "life energy" or property that makes them related to us, generating fear or attraction. It could be the shape of a cloud looking like a dead relative or a gnarled trunk of a tree that suggests it once was human. We are still startled when we see such things, but we no longer react with an inspirited interpretation we once took for granted.

Although science has grown immensely as the major source of our new knowledge of the universe and has created new fields of science that did not exist then, we are still very dependent on (or accept uncritically) these older ways of dealing with the world. Most of humanity practices a religion. These religions may be mutually contradictory, but this does not change the faith of those who believe that this is the world that matters. Even for those who have reduced their religious beliefs to social habits out of conformity to family and community expectations, beliefs in the supernatural abound. Many people have a more sophisticated view of their religions and they accommodate science without feeling threatened by it. Among the six billion inhabitants of the earth, this might be a small minority. Most of humanity is biologically illiterate. These chapters describe that illiteracy.

CHAPTER 2

Living on Automatic Pilot

AGOOD PART OF OUR BEHAVIOR is done without reflection and with a minimum of training. We do not have to learn to breathe or swallow. We are not taught how to sneeze, yawn, go to sleep, or walk. How do we do this? Much of life depends on acts that do not require language or sophisticated thinking or training. Most animals use those skills with a high degree of success. We too are animals, but many people do not like to think of themselves as animals because they feel that they will lose their human dignity and special status if they admit this. This is silly. We do not pity physicians because they learn about all of the animal functions of our bodies. Nor do we seriously believe that being a physician means losing one's human dignity.

Breathing and swallowing may be largely automatic, but we tend to think we are aware of what we see. This too is false, as Sherlock Holmes demonstrated on many occasions to the surprise of his friend Dr. Watson. It is also false to every stage magician who creates an illusion of supernatural events taking place before our eyes. But even simple things that we take for granted are a surprise when a scientist analyzes the process that we think is obvious or simple. A good example of this is our perception of motion. Hold up a finger at arm's length before your eyes and wave it back and forth vigorously. It looks blurred, doesn't it? Now hold that finger again at arm's length, keeping it still, and wag your head, side to side or up and down. Your finger is not blurred. It is held in fixed focus. Yet the path of your finger across the retina of your eye is the same in both cases. Why then do you get two different responses? At least two different parts of the brain are involved in humans and many other animals. The fixed focus while your head is moving has the advantage of keeping a predator or food in view while you are in pursuit. The blurred image of something moving in front of you alerts you to possible danger (or an opportunity to look for food) and you turn your head to shift to a fixed focus.

Human beings as we know them are members of a single species, called *Homo sapiens.* Biologists believe that this "anatomically modern human" arose about 130,000 to 200,000 years ago in Africa and moved out of Africa about 90,000 years ago and spread around the rest of the world. Humans survived mostly on automatic pilot as do most animals that are equipped with such adaptive features as mobility (we can walk and run), frontal vision (we see ahead of us), and the skills to obtain food (in our case, a varied diet of found foods such as nuts, roots, and fruits and captured foods such as fish, birds, and other animals). About 40,000 years ago, our ancestors left records of their artistic skills in the form of cave paintings. About 15,000 years ago, we added the domestication of animals (cats, dogs, cattle, sheep) and plants (cereal grains, especially). About 9000 years ago, the first cities began to develop. About 5500 B.C. in Pakistan (the Harappan or Indus civilization), the first written languages appeared. We know very little about the written history of most of the world's people who lived more than 5000 years ago. We know more about their more ancient cultures because humans have left stone tools and chiseled or scraped evidence of butchering on the bones of animals they ate over tens of thousands of years ago.

One of the things that makes us human is the degree to which we have a culture. Culture is passed down by learning and not through our genes. Our genes make us breathe automatically. Our culture makes us aware of gods, kings, gender roles, parents, strangers, and what is dangerous. Humans have communicated by gesture and language probably as long as we have been a species. Other animals have cultures too, but they are less complex. Apes can use tools to retrieve objects, to obtain food, or to prepare a secure place to rest. They teach their young these cultural skills. No other animal but humans communicates with a written language.

Even without a written culture, humans had developed considerable skills to survive. They used rocks and wooden cudgels to strike down animals for food. They developed wooden lances to thrust into animals. They learned to make covered pits or traps to capture food. They learned to use the skins of animals to make clothing and carrying bags. They learned to use leather strips to tie bundles of wood or edible plants and to tote them back to their camping grounds. They learned to use fire and to make fires as protection, as a means of seeing or keeping guard at night, as a warming glow against cold weather, and as a way of cooking and preserving foods.

What gave humans an advantage over other animals working on automatic pilot was their brain. It is easier and faster to acquire skills by learning than by inherited behavior. The human brain is capable of invention. It is capable of empathy. It is capable of developing values. It is capable of generating ideals to live by. But the specific behaviors from these probably genetic tendencies can be across a huge spectrum of activity—good or evil, desirable or abominable, self-serving or universal. These specific behavioral outcomes are not genetic; they are cultural, learned from mimicry or formal instruction.

How to Survive in the Stone Age

Our species, *Homo sapiens*, we noted, arose about 130,000 to 200,000 years ago. There were other species with the genus *Homo* before us and some of them (such as the Neanderthals) lived on another 100,000 years after we appeared before they became extinct. Most species live about one million years before they become extinct or become transformed through natural selection into something else. We are a young species, with 90% of our potential time ahead of us in our current form and with our current capacities. We humans were largely on automatic pilot (in the sense of lacking most of the attributes of historical civilizations) until we shifted from a Stone Age culture to one that employed the skills of domesticating plants and animals as well as the shift from gathering and hunting to communities that farmed. Hunting and gathering was a great teacher by experience. It taught the use of weapons beginning with throwing stones (and stockpiling them for defense or hunting). It taught skills of finding, trapping, outwitting, and butchering prey and using animal products for human uses. Bones became tools for piercing things, grooming (in the form of combs), and fastening things (such as serving as buttons). They could be shaped into fish hooks, earrings, nose plugs, and ear plugs, or carved into statuettes of animals and human-like objects (perhaps goddesses and gods). Stone chips could be used to slice leather into strips to form thongs and strings. Larger and sharper wedges of stone could be shaped into knives and used to cut leather into clothing.

Many of these acquired skills, invented through trial and error, then became traditions and were taught to children and preserved as part of the culture of Stone-Age-isolated kindreds living in bands. If you think about it, quite a lot of reasoning was involved in this experience-based learning and invention. It takes imagination to see a spread-out hide of a deer as footwear, trousers, a blouse, a belt, or laces. It takes imagination to tie a strip of leather to the notched ends of a sapling and make a bow and to take firm sticks and use them as arrows. It also takes a lot of practice and conscious effort, as well as memory of the aim, pulling time before release, and estimating direction, to become a successful archer and bring down moving prey.

Unlike other animals, humans are rarely on automatic pilot for their truly human skills. No other animal can make such sophisticated tools for so many activities; nor do other animals use shaped tools (e.g., flakes from a hammered stone) to make different tools (e.g., fish hooks from bone). Birds can make sophisticated nests. Ants can make sophisticated communities to hatch their eggs or culture their food. Bees can make a sophisticated hive and even communicate distance and location of floral food sources. Humans have to learn those skills. They are not part of being on automatic pilot.

What distinguishes human uses of tools is the extended habitat they provide. Humans can develop tools for fishing, for hunting, and for harvesting. They can develop tools to cross rivers and to fish in lakes or at seashores. They can migrate for hundreds of miles and find their way back or set up new enclaves in new environments and develop tools appropriate to these new environments.

Humans were limited in Stone Age cultures for skills that require a civilization. They were vulnerable to germs and had no way to effectively prevent infectious diseases from killing their children. They had little control over droughts and bad weather until they learned to build permanent shelters. Caves were safe, but there were not enough of them for a growing human population. No tools were available to create caves from solid rock. It took 50,000 or more years of life in Africa before humans of our species began to move into the Middle East and slowly fan out over the next 30,000 years to Asia and Europe and eventually from Siberia to Alaska and the continents of the Americas.

Recommended Reading

Accounts of early human Stone Age life are abundant. I recommend Steven Mithen's *The prehistory of the mind: The cognitive origins of art, religion, and science* (1996. Thames and Hudson, London).

Between Gods and Beasts

W E KNOW THAT HUMANS BELIEVED in supernatural explanations of their origin and their relation to the universe about 3000 years ago, when the oldest scriptures (often called the Torah or the first five books of the *Old Testament* called the Pentateuch) were written by scholars in a Hebrew civilization. The Book of Genesis reveals the world view of that time. Humans perceived themselves as a distinct creation in the image of that creator, unnamed but referred to as Yahweh or Jehovah. Plants were created separately before animals, and humans were a last-day creation in the 6 days of activity that led to the universe as our ancestors knew it. They also saw the sun, moon, planets, and stars as being created after the earth and plant life were created, a view now impossible to reconcile with evolutionary studies in the life sciences and physical sciences of the twentieth century.

Belief in the supernatural predates written records or Hebrew civilization. We know that some of the caves that date 30,000 or more years ago had altars, that chimeric figures were drawn on cave walls, and that carved figures, especially of pregnant women, were prepared from bone and ivory. We assume, but cannot know, that these were part of a religious system of our distant ancestors. We know that many of these caves included burial grounds with a variety of objects included to accompany the dead. We infer from this (with reasonable likelihood of being correct) that they considered life after death possible. But that other world cannot be seen by the living, and the dead do not come back to sit among us, except in our dreams; so these ancient humans drew up a world of spirits or souls inhabiting that world. By analogy with cultures studied by anthropologists, we also infer that sometimes these dead spirits could be prevailed upon to help individuals or the community. If the dead were killed for transgressions against the community, they needed to be appeased or diverted by other spirits from causing harm.

The World View of the Faithful

Those with faith are often more assertive about their beliefs. With so many hundreds of religions, however, it is clear that no matter how devout members of any one religious group may be, they cannot claim that all religious people believe the same things. In fact, many of those firm believers look upon other religious beliefs as being in error and introduced by Satan (or his equivalent) to lure the less faithful away from salvation. They would prefer that all of humanity worshipped in the same way. We call such true believers fundamentalists or orthodox extremists. They can be found in sects of Judaism, Christianity, and Islam, three related religions that call themselves monotheistic or worshipping a single god. All, to some degree, accept the book of Genesis as the historical record of God's creation of the universe. They differ in the relation of the faithful to that God and to each other in the community of believers. Many other religions are polytheistic with multiple gods. This was especially true in the early civilizations that arose in the Middle East (Sumerian culture and religion), the Nile valley (Egyptian deities), Mexico and Central America, and India (Hinduism). Buddhism and Confucianism were founded by humans as ways to live and not by humans claiming to be deities. Most religions evolve and some die and are demoted to the status of myths. That was true of the two civilizations most influential on European and American culture—the Greeks and Romans, whose numerous gods still influence our poetry, literature, and art.

Faith is essential for those who believe in their own religion and its creedal requirements. Rituals, holidays, and rites of passage are not based on reason but on tradition or revelation. Most of these activities keep a community identity alive and they foster bonds among people who are not immediate kin. Although these provide the benefits of a community, they can also provide a basis for bias (against nonbelievers) and a belief that the supernatural can be invoked to benefit the faithful and punish the transgressors (despite works such as the Book of Job that clearly show that one's relationship to God is inscrutable).

We date the start of modern science to the works of Copernicus, Galileo, and Harvey—the late fifteenth to early seventeenth centuries. They were the first to shatter the world view of the Medieval World, which was heavily influenced by Christianity and embedded in theology. Copernicus was the first to suggest a solar system, shifting earth out of the center of the universe. Galileo was the first experimental physicist to use experiments and tools of science (especially the telescope) to confirm Copernicus and extend our knowledge of the physical universe to include the moon, the planets, and the sun as material objects, rather than perfect spheres in circular orbit around the earth, with all, except the earth, emitting their own light. Harvey was the first to show that the human body acts like a machine—the heart pumps blood. In the last half of the seventeenth century, Isaac Newton profoundly changed our view of the universe and how it worked with the publication of his *Principia Mathematica* in 1687. His view of universal laws of physics extended his equations to the motions of the planets as well as the objects moving on earth.

The shift from a world view before 1500 to the scientific world view that has flowed ever since has been accompanied by denial, resistance, and accusations of heresy against scientists who promoted these views. Copernicus waited until he was in his deathbed before he allowed his book to appear. Galileo had to recant his views. Harvey enjoyed the protection of the King to whom he was his physician. Fortunately for Harvey, the demonstration of the heart as a mechanical pump was compatible with a view of the human body as base and a mere housing for a soul. Among Harvey's contemporaries, the body was still corrupt, temporary, and closer to animals than to the divine. The mind (not yet associated with the brain) was what mattered and it was seen as occupying the body. By the time Newton's theories were published, the world view of humans had changed. God was seen as using natural laws, rather than daily miracles, to make the days and seasons possible.

Recommended Reading

For an overview of the origins of the major monotheistic faiths, I recommend Karen Armstrong's *A history of God: The 4000-year quest of Judaism, Christianity and Islam* (2004. Gramercy Press, New York). An introduction to the rise of modern science is available in Dava Sobel's *Galileo's daughter: A historical memoir of science, faith, and love* (1999. Walker and Company, New York).

CHAPTER 4

Our Negative Image of Our Animal Self

W E TEACH OUR CHILDREN TO MAKE PRIVATE those aspects of our lives that we associate in a negative way with other animals. We defecate and urinate out of sight. We reproduce in the privacy of our bedrooms. We look with disapproval at people who cut their nails in public or who pick their noses. We apologize ("excuse me" or "I'm sorry") if we sneeze or cough and we get disapproving glances if we do so without making an effort to trap our own germs in a handkerchief or tissue paper. In some cultures, kissing in public is forbidden. Most of the industrialized nations do not approve of a mother publicly nursing a child on a train, in a bus, sitting on a park bench, or other public place. We have laws about decency that vary with religious and social custom, including when and where people can walk with parts of their bodies uncovered (beaches are legal, but walking seminude in bathing suit trunks in midtown Manhattan could invite an arrest for indecent exposure). Not all of these customs are inappropriate for their own cultures, but our relaxation of laws and customs do change with time. As humans, we have to act as if we are not animals.

The good reason for our minimizing animal habits in public is that we want to focus on our human side and not on our animal side. That is rational. Denying our animal side is irrational, but forcing others to observe our animal side is usually rude and offensive. We are more observant of that code of behavior with strangers and formal settings than we are in the presence of our immediate family. Parents spend a good deal of time socializing their children so that they will not act like animals in public.

Denying Our Animal Self

I was once at a genetics meeting and my roommate in the dormitory to which we were assigned got on his knees and prayed. I had never seen an adult (he was in his 30s or early 40s) pray at a bedside and found this curious. I assume he felt that this was not a private matter just between himself and his God and that praying in front of a stranger was not improper and served a higher cause.

At one of the sessions of this meeting, a speaker discussed an evolutionary aspect of human behavior and my roommate got up with indignation and said, "I am a human. I have a soul. I am not an animal. Evolution makes me an animal." As is usually the case at scientific meetings, when a religious statement is made in a secular setting, the speaker did not reply and the audience was subdued (with many no doubt considering this person a "religious nutcase").

What struck me was not this person's religious beliefs and strength of piety, but his argument that his soul (not his mind) somehow separated him from animals and an evolutionary past. His view may be unusual for a geneticist, but it is not at all unusual for a substantial portion of Americans and probably of the world as a whole. I suspect that many people are at war with their own bodies because they see this aspect as being animal. We see a spectrum of responses in the history of our attitude toward our animal nature. Besides mortification of the flesh, humans have fasted to chastise their improper thoughts or behavior. They have sought forgiveness for their sexual thoughts or acts. They have tried, mostly for nonreligious reasons that some would equate with vanity, to compensate for their aging by dyeing their hair and using surgery to eliminate their wrinkles, electrolysis to remove hair from inappropriate places, and other cosmetic means to present a more youthful appearance in a culture that values youth and that looks, with fear, avoidance, and dismissal at those who accept their aging animal bodies.

No matter what our religious beliefs and no matter how fervent our desires, we cannot escape our animality. Our metabolisms produce body wastes. Our minds bubble up improper thoughts whether we agree with Freud's interpretations of them or not. Our bodies will age. All the will in the world cannot arrest the consequences to our diminished abilities, lost teeth, failing eyesight, memory losses, painful arthritic joints, and other afflictions of the aging process. We are mortal because we are animals and not gods.

This does not mean that we must celebrate those animal aspects, although our literature is rich in the sorrows of those immersed in their animality, their life cycle crises, and their inept responses to situations most of us learn to take in stride or sublimate in creative ways. But we do celebrate the joys of our youth and our romances and we cultivate our bodies with exercise, sports, and other playful acts. We appreciate our bodies when rendered by artists, when interpreted by dancers, and when we watch spectator sports. For many people, what makes us tick is not just Freud's assessment of "work and love" but what psychiatrist Roderick Gorney calls "work, love, and play."

Appreciating the Human Biology We Do Not See

We share with many other animals, especially our fellow vertebrates, a cellular composition, similar tissues (nerves, muscles, skin, and bone), similar organs (lungs, kidneys, brains, livers, and guts), a life cycle, sexual reproduction, and many behaviors. We are human because we have many differences compared to other animals. We are bipedal and can walk and run using our lower limbs. We can communicate through an elaborate speech that describes the world around us. We are dependent on making and using tools to construct shelter, obtain food, clothe our bodies, and practice a hygiene that protects our health. We share with all life the possession of genes, chromosomes, and a place (the cell) where these molecules can carry out a life cycle. Our knowledge of our molecular composition is restricted to the findings of the last 50 years. Our knowledge of our cellularity is something we have known for less than 200 years. Our knowledge of our heredity is about 100 years old. Much of humanity is still ignorant of every aspect of life smaller than a pinhead. Many people act as if physical agents like tobacco smoke, ammonia, nitric acid, and peroxides that are part of our industrial environment or personal habits have no effect on them because they are ignorant of the way these products act on genes and cells and damage them. Knowledge of our animality gives us a sense of our vulnerability and an opportunity to protect ourselves (and future descendants) from harm.

What It Means to Acknowledge Our Animal Aspects

Whatever one's religious beliefs about the existence of a soul or the mind as something apart from our brain, there is no denial of our mortality. The body ages, has the potential to ail, and we die. These are not the aspects of the body we appreciate. We appreciate our athleticism in our youth and test our skills for skating, biking, running, swimming, and competitive sports. We look upon our young bodies with pleasure and equally so when we observe young adults regardless of our age. The body is fine-tuned to do its work. We also recognize that to keep our body in shape we have to walk, exercise, or set aside time to engage in physical activities if our occupations are largely bound to a desk. As humans, we vary in that commitment. Some cultivate the body and build muscles through considerable exercising with specialized sports equipment. Some set aside time to play tennis or swim as a way to keep the body in shape. Some have no choice because their occupation involves physical labor that is demanding on the body. Similarly, some are so bound to their work sitting down at a desk that they never set aside time to exercise.

We appreciate specialists who study the body as we know it. Physical therapists do wonders for those whose muscles have suffered from disuse. We go to our physicians to restore to health those parts of our bodies afflicted with disease or injury. Those who engage in sports professionally have coaches and physical trainers who improve skills needed for those sports. Some combine religion and the body through yoga, tai chi, and other ritualized activities of the body.

It is evident from this inventory of our habits that we are ambivalent about our bodies and have both positive and negative images of them. We can augment our knowledge of our body through an understanding of its biology. This too will lead to a range of responses from disgust, fear, and denial to stewardship, awe, and delight. There is a major difference between our body and mind dualism at the level of our working bodies and the intricacies of our cellular, genetic, and molecular bodies.

We do not invoke a similar spirit or soul permeating our genes, chromosomes, cells, organelles, and tissues at the microscopic level. That reflects our prior ignorance of life at the microscopic level. Souls and spirits are whole-body phenomena carried over from a world view attuned to our perception of the world without scientific instruments. The one exception to this relative ignorance of our microscopic life is in the area of reproduction. It was not known until the 1870s that fertilization involved the union of one sperm and one egg. When fields such as prenatal diagnosis and in vitro fertilization emerged, a shift to interest in fertilized eggs and early embryonic cells (called stem cells) came into being. This interest does not apply to the somatic cells that are shaved off our bodies or dribbled as blood into oblivion down our sinks. Yet the nuclei of such somatic cells will someday be altered (as they have been in other mammals such as sheep) and serve to produce embryonic stem cells or potential clonal twins. In a sense, if one believes that ensoulment resides in embryonic cells, then it potentially resides also in nuclei of somatic human cells used to make future stem cells that have the capacity to become human twins.

Recommended Reading

There is not as much attention paid by social scientists to our body taboos in western culture. Sigmund Freud, of course, made it a central theme of his psychiatric view of humanity. His *Civilization and its discontents* (1930. The Hogarth Press, London) abounds in such insights.

CHAPTER 5

Mind, Soul, Ideals, and the Ephemeral

MUCH OF OUR VIEW ON WHAT IT MEANS to be human comes not from the Judeo-Christian religions but from Greek philosophic views. We owe to the ancient Greeks, especially from the time of the fifth century B.C. to its replacement by the spread of the Roman Republic, a view of humanity that is dualistic. Not only were the body and the soul separated, so also were mind and matter. In more formal ways, whatever most of humanity looks upon as real (anything shaped by human labor, tangible, or perceived by our senses), many Greek philosophers, especially of the Platonic school, looked upon as corrupt, temporary, and unreal. Rather, what was real was the ideal. In the most abstract presentation of reality, the predecessors of Plato, the Pythagoreans, looked upon mathematical forms such as circles, triangles, squares, pentagons, and other objects as real if they could be described mathematically. Geometry was one such way of depicting ideal (and hence true, real, or permanent) objects.

When I published my book, *The Unfit: A History of a Bad Idea*, a friend of mine who is a Catholic priest and at the time a faculty member at a seminary near Cold Spring Harbor, remarked, "Yes, you can have a history of a bad idea but you can't have a history of a good idea because the good is universal and independent of time. It does not change." I have reflected on his remark and do not agree with his assessment. It is historically clear that our *interpretation* of the good changes. In 1924, it was a good idea to sterilize the unfit because they were perceived as a degenerate set of people who hurt society by their incapacities, physically and morally. The naïve assumptions of the good included, at that time, a belief that heredity was "like for like," with good people producing good children and unfit people producing unfit children (among them, paupers, criminals, psychotics, and the mentally retarded). It also included a belief that a higher good (a healthy humanity) was desirable for contemporary society because the unfit could not cope with such complexity and drained society's resources for their care or isolation. After World War II and the revelation of the Holocaust and other atrocities done by Nazi eugenics, the idea of sterilizing the unfit was perceived as mischievous or evil. Unlike mathematical concepts that have defined axioms and mathematical equations or symbols to express them, the concept of the good in social or religious usage is faith-based and not reason-based and almost certain to generate controversy rather than agreement.

The Denial of the Material World Leads to Confusion and Harm

We live our lives in a real world where we accept as real the objects we recognize with our senses. This includes our own bodies. Shifting the real to some idealized perfection, if not false, is misleading or harmful. It leads to erroneous beliefs that the mind can control material things by sheer will. Many people believe that they can cause harm to others by cursing them, sticking pins in images of them, or finding someone who can cast a spell on another person. Many people also believe that they can see future events before they happen or receive thoughts or visual images of people (usually relatives or acquaintances) and objects as they are happening in other parts of the world. They may believe that they possess a property called luck that will allow them to gamble successfully. If they happen to win a rare event like a lottery, they often believe that they were chosen by God to receive that huge sum of money. Just as the gambler believes in being lucky, those who abuse their bodies with tobacco will reject the scientific basis for its harmful effects and promote a fatalistic view that it is not the carcinogens in the tobacco smoke but bad luck or a predestined fate that determines who will live or die.

Few people today in industrialized nations believe that the ideal is real and that the ephemeral is of no importance. Instead, most people use a dualism with an acknowledged and important material world, an acknowledged body (similar to that of animals), and an independent mind or soul that is housed in the brain. Some equate the mind and the soul and others perceive them as different entities because the mind develops like the body from birth to old age. A baby's mind is not articulate. A senescent adult's mind may also be inarticulate. The soul is considered everlasting, and few people imagine their parents or grandparents going to an afterlife (let us assume it is Heaven) with a soul that is enfeebled by Alzheimer's disease. Nor do they consider that an infant who dies will have a soul that will be inarticulate and frozen in infancy in that afterlife.

The material world is much appreciated in our era because it provides things we like. People enjoy a variety of foods and ways they can be prepared and where they can be enjoyed from one's kitchen to banquet halls and expensive restaurants. People like clothing and usually have more clothing than they need. They see clothing as more than a necessity. Clothing defines status, it plays a role in courtship, and it contributes to our self-image (which can vary from unpretentious modesty to ostentatious overdressing). People also make their homes a reflection of what they consider important. Scholars enjoy lots of books in their homes. Those with affluence, but who have not achieved their success through scholarly effort, may consider expensive furniture, more rooms than they can live in, well-cared-for front yards, and the neighborhoods where they live as symbols of their status and well-being. Few people choose an austere and simplified material lifestyle like the Amish, who reject modern technology and the pursuit of material wealth. In contrast, many who think of themselves as religious celebrate making money and indulging in the same luxuries as those who were once demonized by preachers of the same denomination in the 1920s as "Mammon worshippers," who put the material world ahead of the spiritual one, which they defined through asceticism and simplicity.

Such confusion abounds because mixed messages are absorbed. If you have faith and are observant in many if not most American religious communities today, it is proper to become rich and live that life with expensive cars and sporting a mansion to live in. But it is not good to have "flesh-serving" behavior, especially if it is sexual. Eating well (but not to excess) is good; dressing in sexually attractive ways is bad. Dancing (particularly by the young) is bad if it suggests sexual activity. Drunken behavior is condemned, but obesity is rarely condemned with equal concern. Puritan standards that prevailed before the 1940s used to condemn most pleasurable activities. Today, many of those activities are tolerated or even endorsed by religious leaders. At one time (the Middle Ages), charging interest for loans was considered usury, a sin. Today, hardly a Christian banker would be condemned from the pulpit for charging interest for loans.

I do not single out religion to condemn it. All political and social philosophies of how we should live experience their own sets of contradictions if studied from an historical perspective. Most of us are blessed with a collective amnesia about the past and are unaware of how often and rapidly (from the perspective of centuries or millennia) our world views change. One of the features of being human is that we are diverse in our personalities and interests. What religions and social or political philosophies usually seek is uniformity of behavior and belief. Ideological purity is hard to sustain or achieve and this leads to purges, heresy trials, shunning, excommunication, or even bloody outcomes.

The Problems of Faith-based and
Reason-based Knowledge

For realists, there is no great difficulty in assuming that there is an external reality and that we are alive and real and part of that reality. The confusion occurs when the mind is divorced from the brain and becomes something supernatural. This permits us to entertain ideas of disembodied spirits such as ghosts and to doubt our own existence. If a soul or spirit is not composed of matter and cannot be detected or proven by scientific means, how do we know we exist? It is the stuff of reincarnation and other devices in religion that appeal to us because they offer hope for an everlasting life. No one enjoys the idea of nothingness as an answer to "What is our future after death?" Realists who are atheists or those whose religion does not include a life after death take that "nothingness" stoically.

Philosophers and scientists describe a curious belief that some people have that everything (the entire universe) is a construction of one's own imagination. In its extreme form, nothing exists except possibly you. This is called solipsism. We reject this because we do not think of ourselves as being fantasies of someone else's imagination. In its milder, academic form, it is called postmodernism with alleged scientific theories being social constructs or consensus rather than descriptions of reality. Most scientists overwhelmingly reject both the milder and more extreme forms of subjective construction as a description of their activity.

There is another problem with faith-based and reason-based knowledge. Although some extreme believers of their faith see a 6000-year-old universe created in 6 or 7 days as described in Genesis as true, they do not think this is a matter of faith but a perfectly reasonable conclusion because the Bible to them is an historical document that describes what actually happened. It is to them a real history of events that took place. Some critics of science point out that the reverse is true for science. It is alleged to be faith-based! Their conclusion comes from the inability of scientists to prove that the universe is real (you have to assume it is real and not an illusion or take its existence on some sort of "secular" faith). Those critics also say it is faith-based and not reason-based to say there are laws that are universal to describe the universe and its contents. Science is limited to what it finds and what it can verify by its predictions. It has to take on faith of some sort of belief that there are many more fundamental laws of the universe to be found or that the number of laws of the universe is virtually all known and few new ones will be found in this coming millennium. We also have to have some sort of faith (we call it preference or conviction or calling) that doing science (or any other activity) is worth doing.

There is a difference among these three components of doing science that are claimed to be faith-based and the tenets of particular religions that are faith-based. There are few, if any, tenets that are universal to all religions. Most are parochial in the sense that they belong to Roman Catholics (mass, confession, the role of the Virgin Mary in religious custom), or to Orthodox Jews (the Messiah has not yet come, Kosher laws are essential because they are God's demands of being Jewish, circumcision must be done to the newborn sons), or to Unitarians (each person is obliged to find his or her own meaning in life while being respectful of diversity and seeking a more just world). In general, the faith-based tenets of religions have a spiritual aspect connecting them to a divine being (among Unitarians, this is optional).

Scientists tend to use the assumptions of reality and scientific laws as universal. There is no parochial way of doing science. Attempts to do so, such as the Lysenko movement in the USSR in the 1930s, failed because a state-mandated science (chosen by politics and not by scientific debate and resolution on scientific grounds) is bound to collapse, and during its brief existence, it will be repudiated by the rest of the world's scientific community. Its collapse will come about because wishful thinking by the state cannot substitute for reality. Shattering heredity and retraining it by the environment to change winter wheat into spring wheat in order to produce bumper crops of much needed food may have made logical sense to Lysenko and his followers, but eventually, all scientific theories have to meet the test of their predictions or die. Lysenkoism died.

We like to have everything connected into a mental fortress that is impenetrable. Yet, when we live our individual lives, we recognize that we can never be perfect saints and that our governments can never be corruption-free or free of human venalities. Science is also a human activity. It has its rogues who fake data, steal ideas, or plagiarize published papers. It also has its fallible human activity of doing sloppy or inadequate experiments and leaping to conclusions. Motivations and personalities of scientists are complex and often independent of the quality of the work they do. People you would avoid socially may do Nobel-quality work. People you admire as scientists may never achieve first rank among their peers. What protects science from being rejected as a valid means of interpreting the universe is not its perfection and self-consistency, but its ability to admit that it can be wrong, that its results must be verified by others who repeat it, and that its predictions can be tested by others. Reason-based science demands this self-corrective process by which understanding is won. Religious-based faith does not usually invite questioning of its tenets (a behavior that it often equates with heresy).

Living with Contradictions Requires an Appreciation of Our Biology

Knowledge of our human biology does not usually replace traditional religious, political, or social philosophies. It supplements them. Such knowledge does not lead to conformity, but it does reduce the incidence of erroneous beliefs about the human condition and encourages more reflection about our relationship to each other and to our environments. This is a good thing because relying on our reason, discussing complex issues, and avoiding false or divisive concepts such as racism, nationalism, sexism, or class bias would greatly diminish the damage that we do to each other. Traditional morality has failed to minimize these harmful concepts because either it is unaware of the hidden (and false) assumptions about human nature that foster them or it assumes those assessments of human nature are true. Racism is based on the false belief that the biological differences that set apart different ethnic or racial groups are indicative of different behaviors among these culturally different groups. Nationalism believes that there are specific hereditary components to the cultural values that bind a nation or people together. These are thought of as favorable (for those who enjoy a common heritage) or unfavorable (for those who are not born or assimilated into that culture or people). Sexism exists because people often assume that cultural gender roles are based on a rooted biology in genes or hormones, or both. In those countries where women have the same educational opportunities as men and where women have been successful in breaking down the prejudices or traditions of the past, women have found their mark in politics, universities, the health professions, and virtually all fields once dominated by males. Class bias also is permeated with assumptions that those who are poor, who are stuck in jobs associated with unskilled labor, or who live in substandard housing or neighborhoods are inherently flawed, lazy, stupid, or freeloading on society, especially if they are forced into welfare to raise their children.

We cannot challenge those views on moral grounds alone. What they do have in common is assumed hereditary dispositions for the negative traits associated with those out of favor. To explore those claims and to see what our humanity would be like if their assumptions are shown to be false, we must know enough of our human biology to enter the debate more effectively. The following section discusses our human biology.

Recommended Reading

For a view of the values and beliefs of the first 25 years of the twentieth century, read Frederick Lewis Allen's *Only yesterday: An informal history of the 1920s* (1931. Harper & Brothers, New York).

For an account of how a state took over science, see Nils Roll-Hansen's *The Lysenko effect: The politics of science* (2005. Humanities Books [Prometheus Press], Amherst, New York).

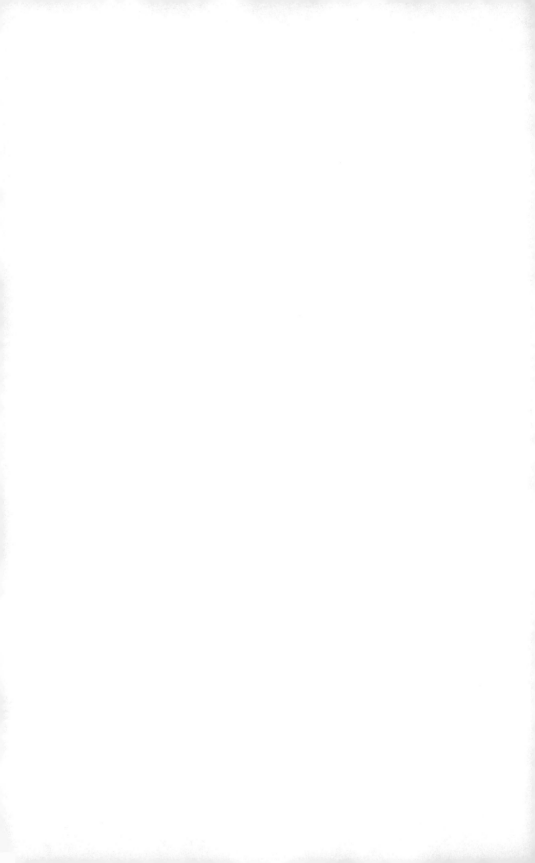

PART 2

Confronting and Recognizing Our Biology

T HE SIX CHAPTERS THAT FOLLOW DESCRIBE what we should know about our human biology. I argue that this knowledge is essential in fields such as medicine and ecology, where an understanding of life enables better health and better stewardship of the world we live in. We begin with the body as a machine, the first biological aspect of our humanity that emerged in the sixteenth century, and continue with the world revealed by microscopy as our cellularity became evident. This quickly applied to a new field of medicine, pathology, which could be used for diagnosis. I then discuss the implications of our having evolved and the kinship this creates with the rest of the living world. Our heredity did not become known on a solid basis until the mid twentieth century, and new fields of genetic services in hospitals have since emerged in response to this flood of knowledge. Also in the mid twentieth century, we shifted biology to a level below the cells and began to understand who we are at a molecular level. That flood of knowledge at the molecular level continues and it has enriched and will continue to enrich and astound us throughout the rest of the twenty-first century because so many more tools are available to make use of this knowledge of our genes.

Two aspects of significance to us (because they go beyond the body) are also included in this section. One is our sexuality and how it emerges from fertilization and leads to baby boys and baby girls. It also throws us into controversy about how our brains respond to hormones in our mother's womb and whether this influences the way we identify ourselves as males or females and the people with whom we are comfortable as sexual beings. Even more controversial are those aspects of human behavior that are not sexual but that define how our personalities are described, our attitudes toward others who are not kin, and the emergence of loyalties to groups. Interpreting these at a cellular, genetic, or molecular level is still far away, but it is beginning. At the organ level, I discuss our brains and what neurobiology teaches us about neuronal functions shaping what we call the mind.

CHAPTER 6

Biology Becomes Mechanistic and Emerges as a Science

T HE CONCLUSION THAT THE HUMAN BODY ACTS as a set of machines is bound to irritate those who have a more dignified view of the human body or even that of other animals. But all life consists of components that work as parts of a machine, albeit an organic one. As thinking humans, we, of course, have to think of ourselves as more than a machine. We act as if we have free will and certainly we make choices, override them, regret them, or celebrate them. We feel a range of emotions that the machines we have contrived cannot experience. It is important to distinguish the body as a machine and the mind that is generated by our neurons in our brain. The mind has enormous capacities for learning, relating, and deciding. These are not activities associated with mere mechanism, at least not at a level that we can presently perceive or imagine. But the body has a structure revealed by studies of anatomy to carry out specific functions and in this way it resembles a machine.

These ideas begin with Andreas Vesalius, a sixteenth-century Belgian physician, who was the first to study human anatomy directly from human cadavers, an act that had to be done in secret because dissecting a corpse was considered a crime. Vesalius's detailed analysis of the bones and muscles of his cadavers revealed how muscles worked and used bones as levers and other tools to perform work. All medical students learn these functions of the muscles in their anatomy courses. Virtually none are converted into atheists by dissecting a human body. Vesalius was a pious Lutheran who lived his faith throughout his life.

The Circulation of the Blood Adds to
the Machinery of the Body

In the seventeenth century, William Harvey performed a number of experiments on veins, arteries, and the hearts of animals and compared this information with what he knew from performing medical procedures on humans. He found that blood from cut veins in the arm revealed the blood to be coming from the portion near the hand and not from the portion near the shoulder. The reverse was true for a cut artery. This suggested to Harvey that blood was circulating, with the heart acting as a pump and sending arterial blood under heavy pressure to all parts of the body. The blood somehow gathered in veins and returned to the heart. Harvey demonstrated this by piercing the ventricle of a deer's heart and showing how blood spurted out when the ventricle contracted. He calculated the volume of blood and how often the blood circulated through the body each day. He noted that veins in the legs contain valves to prevent blood from flowing back toward the feet. Such valves are absent in the arteries.

In 1628, Harvey did not know how the blood returned from the arteries to the veins that brought the blood back to the heart. Some 40 years later, Marcello Malpighi discovered capillaries using microscopes to identify them. Microscopy was not available when Harvey was doing his experiments.

The French Establish Physiology as
an Experimental Science

Chemistry and physics dominated the scientific studies of the 1700s, and science was still seen as compatible with religion. This began to change in France among the scholars who lived a generation before the French Revolution. The idea of an intelligent designer was not yet in vogue, but those who were religious and sought new revelations from "the bible of nature" were not finding much of a religious nature. Instead, they were finding lots of useful applications from their basic sciences and they were adding to the knowledge of how the universe worked. This led to a school of scholars who called themselves deists. They believed that God's role was creating the laws of science. For them, the universe was like a gigantic clockwork machine, whose motions were mathematically described by science and whose contents and future locations could be described with remarkable accuracy. This universe was materialistic because all of the objects in the universe—sun, moon, stars, and planets—were thought by them to be material bodies. Newton's laws of gravity and the physics of static bodies and moving bodies suggested to them that the universe was orderly and governed by laws that humans could use to predict everything from solar and lunar eclipses to the return of comets in their highly elliptical paths.

This secular perspective of science was absorbed by French physicians in the first half of the nineteenth century. They looked upon the body as a machine upon which experiments could be done to reveal its functions. The stomach was shown to be a digestive organ, and hunks of meat and other food were introduced by strings and pulled out at different times to show the process of digestion (the nature of those digestive juices, later called enzymes, was not then known). The pancreas was also shown to secrete digestive juices. The saliva in our mouths was shown to convert starch into sugar. We eat to recycle what we eat.

Physicians learned to use instruments to measure body temperature, to look with a reflecting mirror at the back of our throats, to listen to our heartbeat, to detect murmurs and use these to diagnose pathologies of the heart, and to take our pulse rate. Physicians learned that hands that dissected corpses during autopsies could kill women examined during their pregnancies by medical students and physicians. These very material findings had enormous importance to the understanding of diseases and preventing them. In the past, medicine was limited to vague theories of fluids being out of balance or vague and unidentifiable toxins that needed to be bled out of the body by cutting veins, by inducing vomiting, and by endless enemas purging the lower bowel for these alleged and nonexistent toxins.

God was absent from these findings as motivator or as author writing in a book of nature. The materialistic world that gathered momentum in the nineteenth century disturbed those whose outlook was more spiritual, like Ivan Turgenev, whose novel *Fathers and Sons* describes the reaction of the father whose son returns home with his young iconoclastic medical student friend. When the friend is asked by the son's father what he believes, he replies, "why nothing; I am a nihilist." Turgenev provided the term that sends shudders down the spines of those raised in a spiritual tradition, who want a personal God who is involved in their lives and the day-to-day events of the world. If God is pushed into the deist's remote edge of the universe, that spiritual world is seen as atrophied or destroyed by secular science.

Note that what has changed at this point is an ideology about the universe and not the nature of science itself. Science can work with the pious (Kepler, Vesalius, and Newton fall in that category) and the deist, agnostic, or atheist (many of the scientists in the eighteenth and nineteenth centuries were deists, including Antoine Lavoisier, Claude Bernard, and Charles Darwin). Ideologies are usually faith-based, whether those ideologies are spiritual or secular. Astronomy, physics, chemistry, geology, and biology are fields of science. They depend on reason, observation, experimentation, and objectivity for their success. Judaism, Christianity, Islam, Buddhism, Deism, agnosticism, and atheism are responses to religions that are all faith-based. Democracy, Republicanism, Monarchy, Socialism, Capitalism, and Fascism are chiefly nonreligious, but they are faith-based.

We Are Dependent on Science Despite Our Ambivalence About Its Effects

Who among us would give up the germ theory and return to a world where half our children would die of infectious diseases? Who would want to live in a world today without government-inspected meats, sanitary laws regulating the cleanliness and hygienic practices of our restaurants, or the life-saving and life-lengthening surgeries and medications prescribed by our physicians? Do we really want a pious world stripped of science? This is an invitation to greater risks of death and misery. But if we accept science in our lives, then we cannot prevent scientists from studying cells, genes, DNA, atoms, galaxies, the geological history of our rocks, the distances of our farthest galaxies, or the evolutionary connections of ourselves to our ancestors, human, primate, vertebrate, and earlier. Asking science to discard reason and to settle for faith-based versions of the material world is like a forced conversion, which may intimidate and silence opposition but has not proven to the unwilling convert what can only be accepted through faith.

Each generation finds a way to accommodate its contradictions. Today, almost all educated people accept that our body acts like a machine or set of machines. We accept the heart as a pump, the stomach as a digestive organ, the sperm and eggs we produce as reproductive cells, the neurons as composing our thinking brains, our hereditary traits as products of our genes, infectious diseases as caused by microbes, and alterations of the genes leading to mutations. Few educated people believe that a child with a birth defect, whether Down syndrome or cystic fibrosis, is a punishment from God for an act performed by a parent or a distant ancestor. Few educated people believe that bad air or unbalanced fluids (once called humors) or unspecified toxins are the major causes of illness. Few educated people believe that psychotic individuals are invaded by devils or that the mentally retarded are caused by a parent's youthful masturbation. Our ideas of disease change largely through the replacement of spurious beliefs by those that are subject to the demands of good science—constant examination by new tests and new technologies.

The body can be interpreted as a machine down to the molecular level and this view will not destroy those whose faiths require spirituality in their lives, a personal God to whom they pray, or an afterlife to which they aspire. Only when science is asked to abandon its findings, shore up faith-based beliefs or change its methodology to include faith-based beliefs, is science in conflict with religion. Only when science leaves the realm of reason and tries to establish and justify as objective an ideology of how we should live our daily lives is it inviting conflict with religion. The two systems of knowledge—reason-based and faith-based—will always live in an uneasy coexistence and mutual tolerance at best because they are fundamentally different ways to experience life and the universe. They are neither mutually exclusive nor mutually interpenetrated.

Biology Emerges as a Science

The sciences are both descriptive and experimental. Descriptive science describes those parts of the universe for which a particular field of science has taken an interest. For astronomers, it is everything beyond the earth. For physicists, it is the properties of matter in all its forms—energy, electromagnetism, atomic structure, optics, statics, and dynamics. For chemistry, it is the property of molecules and how they are formed. For geology, it is the rocks of the earth and the forces that shape them, from rainfall to volcanic eruptions. Biology describes the diversity of life, the variations among members of a single species, and the comparative anatomy and physiology of living things. Description may require special instruments of science to help make more accurate and new descriptions. Telescopes and microscopes are such instruments. So are thermometers, centrifuges, electrophoretic apparatuses, lancets, X-ray machines, beakers, distillers, computers, cyclotrons, linear accelerators, radiocarbon dating equipment, and space robots photographing the surface of Mars.

Experimental science is a major part of physics, chemistry, and biology. It is more difficult to do experiments in astronomy because the objects are so remote. There will be lots of experimental work when humans establish bases on the moon and Mars. It is also difficult to do experiments in geology because of the immense size of mountains, volcanoes, oceans, land masses, and similar bodies that are studied. Experimental science tests ideas about the objects being studied.

Sciences can also be distinguished as dealing with universal properties (chemical reactions, the movement of stars, the chemical composition of genes) and historical associations. Historical sciences such as geology can describe what layers of rock reveal about past vegetation and animal life, and what climate was like thousands or millions of years ago. Very similar historical information can be unearthed by archeologists studying civilizations and communities that have long disappeared from historical knowledge. Much of evolutionary studies in the past two centuries depended on studies of the fossil record to work out the history of life on earth. Those have been supplemented by studies of proteins, genes, chromosomes, and genomes. Biology involves three scientific approaches: descriptive biology, experimental biology, and historical biology.

Those whose knowledge of science is nearly nonexistent often assume that if science is not experimental, it is not real science. If this were true, much of what we depend on for our own lives and for our civilization would disappear. Medicine would not be distinguishable from quackery. Astronomy would be no more reliable than astrology. We would be using a farmer's almanac and not modern meteorology to predict the weather.

Most of Biology Before the 1890s Was Descriptive

Jean Baptiste Lamarck was the first to coin the term "biology" in 1802. He believed that this term would permit botanists and zoologists to share what life had in common. Botany was seen before then as a branch of medicine because most of the drugs used by physicians to treat diseases were derived from plant products. Zoology had a more complex history. Many of the animals described until the 1600s were imaginary (such as unicorns, mermaids, and chimeras) and described along with known rare animals in bestiaries. The problem of classification and diversity became acute after the discovery of the New World and by the sea route access to Asia and Africa by European explorers in the fifteenth and sixteenth centuries. As colonies were established around the world, new plant and animal specimens from these continents flooded into Europe. Carl Linnaeus in the mid 1700s provided a system of classifying them that persists to this day. He coined the term "species" (known vaguely since biblical times as a "kind"). He also invented terms for higher categories of animals or plants with each category sharing a number of common features. His original categories were the kingdom, the class, the order, the genus, and the species. Today, we have many other subdivisions. Thus, you are a vertebrate in the phylum *Caudata* because you have a spine. So do snakes, pigeons, dogs, and whales. But insects, snails, starfish, jellyfish, and worms do not have spines. You are a member of the human species and have the name *Homo sapiens*. Linnaeus did not interpret these classifications as having an evolutionary history. He thought in terms of designs shaped by God. He did not have a consistent belief in the fixity of species. Some of his plants, when hybridized, seemed to form new species. This did not suggest to him an evolutionary mechanism, but it did suggest that variation in life was more complex than he had initially thought.

Along with new specimens from around the world came a number of puzzling observations. Animals and plants were not randomly distributed around the world. Each continent had its own collections that differed, sometimes profoundly so, from those of other continents. It was not just climate that was involved. The life on islands differed from the life on continents. The life on mountaintops differed from the life found at its base. Freshwater and saltwater held different types of life. What caused these differences and why were they not consistent everywhere on earth? As we shall see, Charles Darwin used historical biology approaches to working out an answer that tried to make sense of such a bewildering distribution.

Scientists were also interested in life itself. What was living matter? Was it composed of the same stuff as the nonliving world? If so, what made inanimate matter come alive? In 1818, Mary Shelley wrote *Frankenstein, or the Modern Prometheus* (her poet husband Percy Shelley had dabbled in chemistry during his brief stay at Oxford) to reflect on this puzzle. She and her fellow writers knew of some experiments by Italian scientists, such as Luigi Galvani and others, who used electric stimulation from batteries (known then as voltaic Greek piles) on corpses to cause contractions of muscles, sometimes elevating arms or legs to the shock of the experimentalist. Mary Shelley used a less scientific idea for reanimating Dr. Frankenstein's assorted human pieces to bring about a soulless being. Dr. Frankenstein pored over ancient texts to concoct an elixir or "spark" he introduced into the corpse.

Answers to the nature of life did not come from descriptive or historical science. They began to emerge from experimental science. The Germans were the first to try this technique on the cells of early embryos. They called it "developmental mechanics" (in the German, Entwicklungsmechanik), and we would later call it "experimental embryology."

Experimental Embryology Changed How Biology Is Done

There is an historical irony that the beginnings of experimental embryology in the late nineteenth century involved what are today called stem cells. Hans Driesch, a German biologist, found that if he separated the two cells of a freshly dividing fertilized egg of a sea urchin, the two cells would each become an identical twin sea urchin. He used the term "totipotent" to describe such cells. They had the capacity to produce a complete being, healthy and fertile. Other scientists tried this in different ways. Wilhelm Roux found that, in frogs, if one of the cells was obliterated by a hot needle, the other cell went on to form a half embryo. This led to the idea that some species have totipotent stem cells and other species begin to differentiate their cells early in development. Experimental embryology yielded other findings. Some embryos used chemical gradients to bring about change and this could be shown by cutting off a hunk of embryo and switching places with another chunk. This way, embryos with two heads or two tails could be made. Experiments by Hans Spemann and Hilde Mangold showed that some regions of an embryo were more influential in generating a set of organs and these were given names such as "the organizer." The nature of these chemical agents was not known at the time and merely inferred.

Throughout the first half of the twentieth century, experimental biology developed a set of tools to study living material. Cell biologists learned to break cells apart, suspend their components in fluids, and spin them into layers in centrifuges so that the layers could be analyzed for their functions. From such studies, the components of cells were worked out. They also used a tool called paper chromatography to study the molecules present in a particular fluid or layer being studied. These molecules could be sprayed to give a color indicating their presence and then cut out of the paper and isolated for chemical analysis. By such means, pieces of proteins could be sequenced and the structure of proteins interpreted from the set of fragments or spots after a partial digestion of the cleaned-up molecule. Scientists could use radioactive elements to tag proteins and other molecules and follow their fate in activities such as protein synthesis, or the photosynthetic process, or the way sugars are converted into chemical energy in our cells.

Scientists also learned in 1900 that hereditary traits could be studied after they rediscovered an analysis worked out by Gregor Mendel in the 1860s. Mendelism then led to a new field of experimental biology called genetics, and geneticists tied this to studies of cells, especially the chromosomes of the cells that contained these hereditary units. Working it out was laborious and involved many laboratories, but like embryology and cell biology, the great surprises came from experimentation. This stunning flood of achievements in the first third of the twentieth century transformed biology from a descriptive and historical science into a primarily experimental science.

Recommended Reading

The best overview of the history of biology (up to about 1925) is Erik Nordenskiold's *History of biology: A survey* (1928. A.A. Knopf, New York).

An account of Linnaeus's life and work is in Wilfrid Blount's *Linnaeus: The compleat naturalist: A life of Linnaeus* (2001. Princeton University Press, New Jersey).

For the development of cell biology, breeding analysis, reproductive biology, and evolution leading to genetics and modern biology, see my own book, *Mendel's legacy: The history of classical genetics* (2004. Cold Spring Harbor Laboratory Press, Cold Spring Harbor, New York).

CHAPTER 7

The Human Body Is Composed of Cells

THE TERM "CELL" AS IT PERTAINS TO LIFE was introduced in 1665 by Robert Hooke. He cut a thin slice of cork bark and examined it with a compound microscope that he had designed and could magnify an object by less than 100 times. What he saw were a myriad of empty boxes that reminded him of the monks' cells in monasteries. He thought the emptiness of these cells provided a basis for the buoyancy of cork, but he had no insight into cells being the basic unit of living structure. That generalization came much later in 1838, when two biologists, Matthew Schleiden (a German botanist) and Theodor Schwann (a Belgian anatomist), devised what they called the cell theory. Schleiden found that all of the plants he studied were composed of cells. Schwann had found the same to be true for all animal tissues he looked at, including human tissues.

In 1838, there was not much of a technology for the study of cells, but microscopes were getting improvements, including better lenses that overcame the earlier tendency of lenses to produce blurred images and rainbow-like colors around the objects (spherical and chromatic aberrations, respectively). In the late 1850s, the new technique of stain technology and a variety of dyes (some of them synthetic) made it easier to study tissues and cells by selectively emphasizing their components.

It is quite remarkable that in the mid 1800s, Rudolph Virchow was using microscopes on human tissues to prove that cancer was a cellular disease arising from a single cell. Virchow clarified the cell theory of Schleiden and Schwann and observed that all cells arise from preexisting cells;

however, the mechanism for cell division was not yet known. It would take another generation before the quality of work in stain technology allowed scientists to study the contents of the nuclei of cells. In the 1870s, suspicion centered on thread-like objects, or chromosomes, in the nucleus as being significant in the cell division process. A process called mitosis was worked out that showed a very exact distribution of chromosomes from one cell into its two daughter cells. By the 1880s, scientists recognized a constancy of chromosome number for the cells of an organism and a specific chromosome number for a given species. Also in the 1880s, scientists developed a theory that there was a second cell division called meiosis that was restricted to the reproductive tissue of the ovary and testes, reducing the chromosome number by half and generating sperm or eggs. The combination of these gametes, or reproductive cells, at fertilization then restored the total chromosome number for that particular organism.

What is striking about this knowledge in the late nineteenth century is that for the first time, humans had an understanding of how they came into being. Semen was not some vague influence imprinting itself on a passive lump of female matter and generating life. Reproduction involved two cells and equal contributions of chromosomes by the male and female reproductive cells. This changed our thinking about the gender roles assigned to males and females. Each contributed equally to the offspring. Older ideas from Aristotle into the early nineteenth century believed semen was a fluid or essence. Eggs, in that ancient view, were without form or life and served as a nutrient for the spiritual "homunculus" or essence introduced by males.

What distinguishes the human we know from literature, history, and culture from the human we know by science is technology, the application of scientific knowledge. Without the technology of science, we would not know we have cells. We would not know there are sperm and eggs that we produce. We would not know of the existence of stem cells and their totipotency. We would have no idea of how life works. From the time *Homo sapiens* came on the scene as a species until relatively recently, humanity has lived in scientific ignorance about life. A long cultural tradition provided knowledge. We were alive because we were activated or inhabited by a spirit or soul. The body was composed of dust, taken from the earth, with life that was first breathed into it by a creator. When we die, we return to dust. Once human life arose, it was thought to be perpetuated by males impressing that life into the menstrual blood or unseen material thought to be in a woman's womb. It was all wrong. But who could tell without science, without the instrumentation to reveal nature to human reason?

Cells Have Organelles with Specific Functions

Cells are the basic structural and functional unit of life. Many organisms, such as bacteria, amebas, and blue-green algae, consist of only one cell. Higher organisms are more complex and they consist of large numbers of cells. As organisms become more complex, the cells are organized into tissues, and the tissues are organized in organs. A human being contains 100 trillion cells, but we cannot see a single one of them with our unaided eyes. The existence of cells changed our perception of the structure of the body. The origin of each individual person from a single cell changed our perception of the human life cycle. It made it possible to study our developmental history before birth.

Most cells, including our own, are composed of a large mass of material called the cytoplasm and a smaller mass called the nucleus. Within the nucleus are the chromosomes, most of the time spun out like unwound cotton thread from a spool. The cytoplasm is a collection of membranous organelles embedded in a fibrous and liquid matrix. The outermost organelle is the cell or plasma membrane, which is alive and not just a wrapping, like skin around a sausage or hot dog. The cell membrane uses energy to move molecules into the cell and pour other molecules out of the cell. It is protective and prevents unwanted molecules from entering. It can patch up its minor tears and worn-out parts. Most of it is composed of fat molecules, into which are embedded many proteins that act as channels, or passageways, for the movement of ions like sodium, potassium, and chlorine. If mutations lead to defective channels in the cell membrane, disease can result, such as the common hereditary disease cystic fibrosis. Children born with this condition have a defective chloride ion channel that impedes the movement of chlorine into and out of the cell. Cystic fibrosis is a disease that can be interpreted at a molecular level because science learned how to isolate cell organelles and examine their molecular components and show how they work in normal and pathological states.

The bulk of the cytoplasm is filled with an organelle called the endoplasmic reticulum. This is where protein synthesis takes place in the cell, using instructions that are brought from the genes in the nucleus. These proteins manufactured in the endoplasmic reticulum are stored in another organelle, the Golgi bodies, and then are used to make more organelles or repair them and to do many other jobs in the cell, including signaling and acting as enzymes.

Also present in the cell are organelles called mitochondria, which resemble bacteria in size and shape and probably arose in our very distant evolutionary past as a symbiotic joining of early cells and a bacterium. Mitochondria take simple sugars and convert them into carbon dioxide and chemically stored energy. When you breathe in air, the oxygen goes into your hemoglobin molecules of your red blood cells and gets dumped out into other body cells and picked up by their mitochondria. The chemical energy produced in the mitochondria, stored mostly in molecules called ATP, or adenosine triphosphate, is used to split molecules in the cell into smaller pieces or to stitch smaller molecules into larger ones. Mitochondria are also unusual in having their own genes, about 60 of them. These genes produce many of the proteins in mitochondrial membranes and most of the enzymes involved in converting small molecules into energy-bearing ATP molecules.

In addition to the mitochondria, endoplasmic reticulum, and cell membrane, the cytoplasm contains structures called lysosomes. These are tiny sacs of enzymes that carry out digestive functions in the cell. They digest the worn-out parts of organelles and recycle their contents in the cell. If such enzymes are defective or missing because of gene mutations, then lysosomal disease occurs, including exotic disorders such as Tay-Sachs syndrome, Hurler syndrome, Fabry syndrome, and about 70 other such conditions.

One of the great difficulties scientists face when trying to converse with those in the humanities is the unfamiliarity we have for the unseen components of our bodies. We do not see cells, chromosomes, genes, mitochondria, or cell membranes. We do not see molecules of any kind. Thus, science becomes a foreign language with strange words that are unrelated to human experience. Its processes are understandable to scientists but utterly divorced from human experience. We take great pains teaching our children to avoid matches, knives, broken pieces of glass, and other objects that can hurt them. We see them. It is easy. But how do you teach a child to avoid agents that induce mutations affecting later generations of children? How does one teach a child to avoid agents that act as carcinogens and induce cancers?

By using the tools of science to work out how the body and the universe function and how those findings relate to health, understanding, and an appreciation of ourselves in the universe provides us with a proven torrent of information that is repeatable, reason-based, available to all nations, all religions, and all ethnicities, males or females. It is universal knowledge that does not require acts of faith or luck to find knowledge and apply it. The two agencies that prevent us from assimilating this scientific knowledge are our tradition of living in the familiar universe of our five senses and our tradition of seeing the sciences as separate from the liberal arts of our education. We give to specialists knowledge that should be digested, translated, and incorporated into our being from the time we grasp our mother's knees in infancy until we die of old age.

Our Common Humanity: What It Means to Know Yourself at a Cellular Level

When Walt Whitman said "I contain multitudes" in his song of himself, he alluded to the humanity around him that he had absorbed and the triumphal feeling of being at one with his fellow Americans. We love the humanities because those poetic insights stir our own feelings of awe. As a scientist, I feel similarly in a state of awe knowing that I contain multitudes (perhaps as many as 100 trillion cells) and that their diversity as components of my tissues are coordinated within me to make me aware of myself. It gives me immense pleasure to know that half my mother's chromosomes and half my father's chromosomes reside in me and that in this biological way they are part of me. It gives me pleasure to know that my genome is unique and possessed by no other person. At the same time, I take pleasure in having the same number of chromosomes, the same number of genes, and a universally identical way of using the oxygen I breathe in, the carbon dioxide and water vapor I exhale, and the common machinery of metabolism as all other normal people on our planet. It is a common humanity at our cellular level. At the microscopic level, there are no races, ethnicity, or other distinguishing features of our individuality. At most, we can look at other people's cells and determine whether they are males or females because our sex is determined by two of our 46 chromosomes. Even that is a thrill because a cell is otherwise sexless in its appearance. We can disguise our sex with clothing and other artifices, but we cannot disguise our chromosomes.

Also as a scientist, I can see the value of that knowledge as I celebrate my cellularity. It gives me the opportunity to figure out the causes of disease. It gives me an insight into protecting my cells from harm. It forces me to look outside my body and into my environment. It makes me aware of the pesticides, herbicides, additives, chemical wastes, and radiations that enter my lungs, wend their way through my guts, and permeate my cells, breaking chromosomes here and there, altering genes here and there. Every time I see a smoker, I see a cloud of carcinogens descending on that person's tissues, dribbling anthracenes, peroxides, aldehydes, nitrous acid, and dozens of other known agents that mutate genes and break chromosomes in the cells lining the trachea and bronchial tree. As the smoker inhales in satisfaction and smoke rings form in aesthetic pleasure, I see those epithelial cells lining the trachea bathed in those chemicals, flattening out from the toxic assaults of one cigarette after another, heaping into dead and dying layers; and buried below them the occasional induced tumor cell that will slowly divide by relentless doubling every 3 or 4 months; and 10 or more years later, it will emerge as a marble-sized tumor that will leave the smoker struggling for air. I feel like Mephistopheles watching Faust squander his talents in the pursuit of new and noxious experiences. I also feel like a disappointed guardian angel, unable to influence the material world around me.

Recommended Reading

George Gamow's books are still valuable in giving those with little or no knowledge of science, a view they can understand. I recommend *Mr. Tompkins learns the facts of life* (1953. Cambridge University Press, United Kingdom) for a tour of the human body with Mr. Tompkins reduced to the size of a cell exploring a human body.

CHAPTER 8

The Body Evolves

EVERYTHING HAS A HISTORY. EVERYTHING EVOLVES. Virtually nothing remains constant in the material world. Mountains are turned into sedimentary layers of rocks as ice and other weathering processes crack off small hunks here and there over millennia. Cities rise and fall and the familiar neighborhoods of our childhood sport new buildings with new occupants and new stores. We grow up. Careers change. I am old enough to have worn knickers to school when I was a boy. I filled inkwells in the desks of my classes. I rolled up balls of tinfoil (not aluminum foil) from discarded cigarette packages during World War II. As we go back in time, there is less of the past to see. My mother-in-law, Florence Dawald Miller, has the Civil War canteen of her husband's great-grandfather, Israel Dock Johnson, from Fulton County, Indiana, who survived a Confederate prison camp by eating the raw sweet potatoes he dug up. His brother, Asbury Johnson, was not so lucky; he was killed. The only remnant of her Revolutionary War ancestor, Andrew Babcock, is a piece of the great chain he helped forge and which stretched across the Hudson River to prevent the British fleet from moving up to Canada. Most of her ancestors between those two wars have left no artifacts for her to display. There is an old girl's shoe that her grandmother wore, and a tin toy locomotive her father played with as a boy in the 1880s. Most of what I know of her relatives is from her genealogical searches taken from public records of births, deaths, and marriages. They are names with few stories left behind of what they did, what their personalities were like, what their personal miseries and triumphs were. It is the fate of most of us as we are buried into oblivion by time. I do not know the name of a single person who lived in the sixth century C.E. (Common Era). No one knows the name of a single individual who lived 8000 or more years ago except as revealed or inferred by using a faith-based history in the Old Testament.

What we take for granted about history and our family histories we sometimes find difficult to accept for the longer view of time of scientists. A popular calculation of the seventeenth century put the origin of the universe about 7000 years ago. It was based on estimated ages of births and deaths of the succession of all individuals mentioned in the Old and New Testaments, from Adam and Eve to somewhere in the second to fourth centuries C.E. when the last of the New Testament books was written. Some people accept that today as historically true. Most people, many of them pious, do not. Scientists today use a variety of tools to date the past. They measure the decay of carbon-14, a radioactive element found in the air we breathe and the food we eat. After a living thing dies, the amount of carbon-14 slowly gets converted to carbon-12, losing about half of its carbon-14 every 5000 years or so. Ancient wood can be dated by carbon-14, and such woods are found in long-buried villages of our ancestors who lived before histories were written. Radioactive uranium is used to date older rocks; here, the uranium is converted into lead and its ratio to uranium is calculated to indicate the passage of time. Geologists can calculate the age of sedimentary layers of rocks by counting the number of layers laid down by annual melting of the winter's snows and the deposits of sediments carried by rivers. They can use tree rings and work their way back to more than 10,000 years from the various ancient wood that they have unearthed in a particular area.

Astronomers use the change in the wavelength of light associated with velocity as objects move away from us (producing a red shift) or toward us (forming a blue shift). Very distant objects in the universe are called galaxies. It was noted by Edwin Hubble in the 1920s that the galaxies he observed, no matter where he turned his telescope, were moving away from us (that is, from our Milky Way, which is our galaxy). The universe appeared to be expanding. The red shift can be related to time, and that time is measured in a distance called the light-year. One light-year is the distance covered by a beam of light as it moves from here to wherever it will be a year from now, which turns out to be about

6 trillion miles. Stars are separated from one another, usually by a few light-years (if they are very close to the sun) or by tens of thousands of light-years (if they are a good distance away from our sun in our Milky Way). It would take 100,000 light-years to go from one end of the Milky Way to the other. The nearest galaxy to us, Andromeda, is about 2.5 million light-years from us. Very distant galaxies are about 12 billion light-years from us. These measurements tell us that the universe is very big and contains billions of galaxies; each galaxy contains billions of stars.

Scientists who absorb this knowledge have an appreciation of how insignificant we are in the totality of the universe. It is a humbling thought. At the same time, it is an opportunity for celebration. We are lucky enough to be on a planet that supports life. It is highly unlikely that life exists in the other planets of our solar system, although bacteria-like life might have arisen on Mars before that planet became too stripped of its atmosphere to sustain it.

Life on Earth Has Evolved

Evolution is largely a historical and descriptive science about the history of life on the earth. In the twentieth century, it also became an experimental science. Good science makes predictions that can be tested. Evolutionary science has done that quite successfully and in abundance. Evolution ran into opposition by those who found its contradictions to faith-based belief unacceptable. This was not the first time science ran into that opposition. Copernicus and Galileo experienced that opposition for Copernicus's solar theory and Galileo's telescopic evidence that the earth is the third planet in orbit around the sun. Today, that is not a troubling thought for even the most devout fundamentalist. Times change. Attitudes change. Theologies change. Things evolve.

The evidence that evolution has taken place was proposed by Charles Darwin, who got the idea about 1838 as he sorted through his collections and notes from his round-the-world voyage on the *HMS Beagle*. He noted the following relations: Living things are diverse in kind, and their distribution in the continents and islands he visited was not identical. What caused this lack of uniformity of distribution? A thinking person would entertain several ideas. It could be a random sampling of how they got dispersed from a common site of origin. This could fit a dispersal of life from Noah's Ark and that would be enough to keep a pious person satisfied. It could be related to climate. We know that animals in very cold climates tend to have white fur and that animals living in a dense and varied vegetation tend to have stripes, or spots, or blend in to their surroundings. For the pious, this could be interpreted as God's wisdom in making everything adapted to its environment. Such a view is called natural theology and it was championed in the early 1800s by William Paley. Today, its supporters would call it intelligent design.

Darwin certainly entertained those possibilities, but his data told him that there was more to it than these two sweeping generalizations. One problem was associated with island biology. The islands off West Africa, such as the Azores and the islands off Ecuador, the Galapagos, were both near the equator and roughly about 500 miles from the continents they faced. They were both volcanic islands and had similar climates, yet their animals and plants were totally different. The life on the Azores resembled African animals and plants. The life on the Galapagos resembled western South American life. If it was just distribution, why were the species different from (yet somehow related to) the continental forms? If it was just climate, why weren't the living species alike in both sets of islands? When contradictions occur in science, we have to modify our theories or look for other theories to make sense of everything presently known.

Darwin also had more puzzles to relate. He noted that many of the animals studied by naturalists on the north side of the Amazon River differed from those on the south side of the Amazon River. The birds were the same on both sides of the Amazon. This suggested that the river acted as a barrier to migration for land animals but not for birds that could easily fly across. When he was in Argentina, he noted unusual sloths in the trees, and when digging in the soil, he came across the bones of extinct giant sloths. Why were the fossils related to these living forms? Was there once an ancestral form of this species that lived eons before from which these present sloths descended? It was not limited to the sloths in the area. It was also true for the armadillos in this area. Neither sloths nor armadillos are animals you expect to find wherever you look. Darwin was also bothered by the lizards, tortoises, and birds he found on the Galapagos. The birds were identified by specialists when he came back as new species. Yet they were related to species found in Ecuadorian jungles. It was as if a solitary species from Ecuador had gotten to the islands in some distant past and then fanned out to the different islands adapting to the food and circumstances on each island. Some developed beaks for eating cactus, some for bugs, some for small seeds, and some for large nuts. Was it possible that they did arise from one species and then evolved into numerous species over long periods of time?

Darwin may have convinced himself that evolution had occurred, but he needed a theory, or framework, for the facts that he determined, to account for all of these events and processes. He called his theory natural selection. He chose the term because everyone was familiar with domestic selection. New breeds of dogs, cats, sheep, cattle, pigs, finches, and numerous flowering plants emerged in the nineteenth century as farmers and hobbyists enjoyed breeding animals and plants and looking for useful or attractive novelties. Selection works. Cattle can be made to produce more beef and less fat, chickens to lay more eggs, roses to be more redolent with their sweet scent, and apples to be sweeter, snappier, or tarter. Domesticated selection showed that variations are abundant and that by selection, many varieties can be isolated.

But can nature do what humans do? Darwin argued that it does, all the time. He showed that there are more offspring produced by animals and plants than can be sustained even by good environments. He got that idea from the English demographer and political economist Thomas Robert Malthus. Darwin showed that variation was natural and abundant in every species. He got this evidence by studying barnacles (for 8 years) and was so good at classifying them that he could tell where a specimen given to him had been collected within 50 miles no matter what continent or island it came from.

The difference between a trained scientist's observation and a lay person's knowledge of the same thing can be quite striking. I remember when I was a graduate student first learning to classify fruit flies for their sex traits and body features and mentioned some of my difficulties to my sponsor, Hermann Muller. He told me that once you knew an organism like a fruit fly very well, you could spot subtle features such as bent, split, or shorter bristles on its back. "It's as if you walked into a group of students and one student was missing a nose. You would notice it immediately." He was right. Fruit flies are about one eighth of an inch in length and I could (and still can) identify a fruit fly settling on my finger as a male or a female without the use of a lens.

Darwin's theory of evolution by natural selection argued that natural variations were tested by a diversity of environments. We know that there are hard times with a scarcity of food and good times with an abundance of foods; there are catastrophic events such as floods and droughts, and normal and repetitive changes of the seasons. There could be competition from other species seeking the same foods or breeding grounds. There could be predators around that pounce on the feeble, the straggler, the bewildered, and the less swift. Darwin argued that this did make a difference. Those who are better skilled, with better metabolism, with more effectively coordinated anatomy, with better senses, or with a coloration that makes them less apparent among others in a crowd, are more likely to live and reproduce. They are also more likely to pass on those traits that favored their survival. Note that this assumes that many of the traits associated with a species are inherited rather than acquired by chance. Coloring is inherited. What enzymes digest what molecules and how effectively digested foods are recycled or stored is inherited. What lengths of bones are present or firing time of muscle fibers is inherited. The acuity of the senses is inherited.

Darwin spoke of the abundance of variety in a species, but he did not know the source of that variation or what caused new variations to arise. It took another 50 years after he published *The Origin of Species* (1859) for scientists to identify units of inheritance that were called genes and a process, spontaneous mutation, that led to new varieties of genes.

Human Evolution Relates Us to Ancestral Apes

Darwin carefully omitted human evolution in his book *The Origin of Species*. He knew that it would be controversial enough just to get his theory of natural selection launched as a mechanism for evolution. He was right. A storm of controversy greeted its publication. Darwin kept from the public debate, and he depended on his colleagues, with whom he had corresponded over the years, to defend his theory. Most scientists were convinced by the evidence in Darwin's publications, and by a flood of publications that followed, that evolutionary biology was a legitimate field of science and that natural selection was its most likely interpretation. Eventually, Darwin published *The Descent of Man* and provided his evidence for human evolution. Most of it was based on comparative anatomy with the primates and similarities of their emotions. The only known human fossils at that time belonged to skeletal remains found in

Germany, known as Neanderthals (today called *Homo neandertalensis*). In the 1890s, a second form of human fossil was found and given the name Pithecanthropus (today called *Homo erectus*).

In the twentieth century, intermediate forms that were ape-like in brain volume and facial features (but with teeth less ape-like) were found in South Africa. The genus *Australopithecus* is given to this ancestral form. It was an ape that walked erect like humans. Kenya and Ethiopia have yielded many *Australopithecine* ancestors and early *Homo* ancestors. What is characteristic of these early forms of *Homo* is a shifting from large canine teeth to smaller canines and a shift in tool-making skills. Most important is the increase in brain volume in these ancestors of our species.

Our teeth shifted from eating plants (apes are primarily vegetarians) to eating meat. Eating meat shifted the evolution of our guts and they became smaller than those found in apes. Humans also learned to cook food and the charred remains found in campsites show that cooking was done by these early ancestors (charred bones that had been butchered with the stone tools). Cooking food also leads to smaller guts because it is easier to digest. To obtain game, our ancestors developed something apes cannot do—endurance running. We can run a marathon. Apes cannot. Humans could run antelopes to exhaustion and collapse, even if antelopes were swifter because the antelopes have no metabolism for endurance running. We have bigger buttocks than apes because those muscles are developed for endurance running. The hole in our skull where the brain and spinal cord meet has shifted from the periphery (in apes) to the middle of the base of the skull (in our species), and these early *Homo* fossils show that shift. This permits our head to stay erect, rather than lean forward and toward the ground, when we run or walk.

Human Evolution Is Not Limited to the Fossil Record

Human evolution became molecular when protein and DNA analysis allowed these molecules from some fossils to be sequenced, as the DNA of tissue in the teeth and bones may last many tens of thousands of years. There are two types of DNA available for analysis. One is present in the DNA of mitochondria, the organelles that provide the energy for our bodies. Mitochondrial DNA, we noted, has about 60 genes. The rest of our DNA is in the nuclei of cells and there are about 25,000 genes in humans. Over thousands of years, even in relatively dried-out sedimentary layers, such DNA will degrade into smaller fragments. It is easier to work with mitochondrial DNA because there are dozens or hundreds of mitochondria per cell. From such studies, the bones of Neanderthals tell us that they are a separate species. Their sequences of DNA differ significantly from any sequence found in *Homo sapiens.* At one time, Neanderthals looked like a variety of *Homo sapiens,* but the DNA evidence is clearly at odds with this. As Neanderthal remains are unearthed and some of the bones or teeth yield nuclear DNA fragments, an inventory of Neanderthal DNA is being maintained and compared to our own sequence of genes. Before this century is over, there will be close to a complete genome sequence of our Neanderthal ancestor. No such fossil DNA exists for *Homo erectus*, but if the recently found *Homo floresiensis* in Indonesia turns out, as presently claimed, to be a midget species of *Homo erectus*, then such specimens may yield both mitochondrial and nuclear DNA for assembling a *Homo erectus* genome. The *Homo floresiensis* specimens presently unearthed are about 18,000 years old.

As in all new findings of science, the claims have to be checked by other investigators and new findings to rule out other interpretations. As we noted, science is inherently tentative and must yield to new knowledge and interpretation when the evidence demands it. Faith-based belief is lacking in such humbling humility. It assumes an eternal truth for its beliefs.

While critics of evolution have focused on the fossil record or the chemical and physical dating of fossils, an entirely new approach has emerged from the Human Genome Project. This effort has sequenced the entire set of 25,000 genes in a human sperm or egg. It has also led to the sequencing of the chimpanzee genome and genomes of many dozens of animals, plants, and microbes, leading to a new field of science, called comparative genomics. What is remarkable in this very new field is the correlation of genome evolution with the phylogenetic trees previously established by comparative anatomy. Also startling is the abundance of minor changes in sequence among related species (such as one dozen species of the genus *Drosophila*, the fruit fly). These can be shown by computer analysis to have arisen in a unique sequential branching pattern that confirms one predicted for the evolution of these species by more traditional approaches in the mid twentieth century.

When Is Evolution a Predictive Science?

Charles Darwin was the first to do experiments to test his theory of evolution. He soaked seeds in saltwater and then planted them after having spent several months in a submerged state. A few of the tropical seeds he tested germinated. This showed that it was possible for branches with animal hitchhikers to drift after storms and move from Ecuador to the Galapagos Islands and colonize a few of their animal and plant species in this new environment. Severe storms are not unusual and rafting of insects and small mammals by driftwood is well known in studies of the repopulation of islands denuded by volcanic eruptions (like Krakatoa). Natural processes can lead to distributions to favorable places to reestablish a presence or to be the first of its kind to reach such a new location. It suggested to Darwin and other naturalists why island life often involved smaller-sized animals and a paucity or absence of freshwater-dependent animals such as salamanders and frogs. Seawater would probably kill such animals rafting across several hundred miles on a tangle of tree limbs.

Geneticists were among the first to put evolution to experimental tests. Geneticists ruled out alternative theories of how evolution works. One of these was the belief that the environment alters heredity in a directed way. Thus, cave animals such as fish are often albino and lack eyes. Yet, tests of organisms such as fruit flies grown 69 generations in the dark (equivalent to about 1700 years in human time) produced no change in the fly's response to light or to the pigment of its eyes (still a deep red). Biologists also noted that two or more millennia of circumcision had no effect on the length of foreskin in baby boys. Each generation of Jews has to be circumcised anew. By crossing fish that are blind and albinic with a related species in streams near the cave that has both pigmentation and eyes, scientists have isolated the gene differences between the two forms. A single gene is involved in albinism. About a half dozen genes are involved in the repression of eye formation. It is advantageous in a cave environment for albinism to be selected and for eyeless mutations to be selected because they conserve energy, and in the case of eyelessness, they also reduce infections. There are also gene mutations not present in the fish outside the cave that are selected inside the pitch black cave environment for detection of cave wall surface by water pressure. The fish know where they are through this sensory system and scientists have isolated some of the genes involved. The expectations of evolutionists were supported by the genetic evidence for these inferred gene differences in function.

Geneticists have also tested species formation by a variety of chromosomal mechanisms in plants. By crossing two different species of wheat that grew in Russia and Siberia, geneticists obtained a new species that could not breed with the other two forms and only with its own kind. But this new form turned out to be the same as a species found in North America, and when that form was crossed with the new Russian hybrid species, it turned out to be genetically compatible in breeding and chromosome number. This suggested that the Russian hybrid species made it across Siberia to the New World at some distant past and that form flourished here but became extinct in Siberia.

In the genus *Oenothera*, a group of plants (popularly called the evening primroses) that originated in the New World and that have been cultivated (and become feral) in Europe since they were introduced in the sixteenth century, a very unusual evolutionary mechanism arose in which chromosomes were broken and rejoined to form rings of chromosomes. These ring chromosome complexes make it difficult to sort out genes and new mutations tend to accumulate, some of them acting as lethals to the offspring when they are brought together as common rings from the two parents. Ralph Cleland, the twentieth-century botanist and geneticist, spent his career studying the evolution of these plants and predicted the existence of about 25 varieties or species that should exist based on their assumed chromosome configurations. Eventually, all of these were found and their chromosomes confirmed his predictions.

Scientists have also predicted that living birds like the chickens we eat have the genes for making teeth (which are absent in birds but not in their fossil reptilian ancestors among the dinosaurs and related forms). This suggested an experiment. If a piece of embryonic jaw tissue from a chicken is grafted onto a developing jaw of the mouse, what happens? The mouse produces hen's teeth, reptilian rather than mammalian. To the scientist, this suggests that the gene or genes for this developmental process were silenced or permanently shut off in the chicken. The presence of those signals from functioning genes in the mouse allowed the chicken tissue to express those genes and produce teeth of their dinosaur ancestors.

I expect many experiments to take place as the genomes of apes, monkeys, and humans are worked out and compared. Isolating the genes associated with our humanity will be very exciting. Some of those genes will deal with the anatomical and physiological changes associated with bipedalism—walking and running on two feet. Some of those genes will involve our metabolic differences in how we digest and store our foods. Some will be associated with the visual acuity and coordination that allows us to throw a rock (or a ball) at close to 90 miles per hour and strike a target (such as a catcher's mitt) some 90 feet away. Professional pitchers have been clocked at even faster speeds. Still other genes will be associated with how we think, store our memory, convert visual images into mental images, and relate these to a myriad of associations acquired in an active lifetime. Testing these in mice and other animals will require some ethical forethought, but some may turn out to have medical use and restore functions in those who are mentally retarded or whose behavior is poorly coordinated (as in some cases of cerebral palsy).

Recommended Reading

A superb introduction to evolutionary biology is David Quammen's *The song of the dodo: Island biogeography in an age of extinction* (1996. Scribner, New York).

CHAPTER 9

Most Human Traits Are Determined by Genes, Which Are Composed of DNA

To WADE THROUGH THE MORASS OF CONFUSION and controversy about what is innate and what is acquired, we first need to know what we are talking about. Your body, including its cells, organelles, and assorted molecules, is the product of about 25,000 or so genes that were present in duplicate at the time you were a fertilized egg. This is the "biological you." It is determinism all the way, with relatively little exception, and that is why identical twins (who share a common genotype but who arose from a single act of fertilization with one egg) look like spitting images of each other.

The "cultural you," whether biologically an aspect of your neurons in action or some sort of imagined but faith-based and unprovable soul or spirit or "everlasting you" that will survive your death, is more complex. Some of your behaviors are innate; some may arise from a genetic tendency (but not a specific cultural form), and a huge amount of who you are and how you behave is cultural. This means that you learned it, directly or indirectly, just as you learned your first language, your feelings for the country to which you pledge your allegiance, and whether you love or hate the New York Yankees.

When Hermann Muller in 1926 wrote a paper called "The Gene As the Basis of Life," he meant that the biological inventory of traits in all living things from viruses to humans was a consequence of the activities of genes. No other molecule had the unusual property of copying itself as well as copying its errors. That, to him, was the feature of the gene that made evolution possible. A gene can pass on its mutations, and if they work to the benefit of the offspring, they survive. If the offspring leaves no issue by reason of sterility, death, or other disabling aspect of its capacities, then those genes bite the dust. They do not evolve.

How Are Traits Inherited?

In 1900, the work of a Czechoslovakian monk, Gregor Mendel, was rediscovered by three European scientists. They confirmed that the work he did with garden peas in 1865 could be repeated by them, and they extended Mendel's results to about 20 more species of plants. Soon, those Mendelian traits were reported for animals (chickens and mice) and then for humans. In 1903, a graduate student at Columbia College, who was studying chromosomes in grasshoppers, Walter Sutton, came up with an interpretation that brought together two fields of science. He said Mendel's genetic ratios were predictable from the behavior of chromosomes that moved during a cell division process, meiosis, which led to the formation of sperm or eggs. He called this the chromosome theory of heredity.

Mendel found two laws. One of them applies to a pair of related traits. The traits are related because they exist as two forms of a common gene. In human terms, think of this as an albino and a person who has normal pigmentation of the skin and hair. One form of albinism involves an absence of an enzyme called tyrosinase. Tyrosinase is needed to stitch together molecules of tyrosine. Tyrosine is an amino acid, and it is abundant in meat and in plants that are high in protein, such as legumes. When tyrosinase binds together strings of tyrosine, a molecule is formed that is called melanin. Melanin is made in specialized cells of the skin and that melanin is stored in other skin cells and gives individuals their particular skin color. In humans, this can be very pale like Scandinavians, tan like Mediterraneans, a bronze color as is present in much of China, Japan, or native Americans, or a range of brown to black skin colors in the Middle East, South Asia, Australia (among the aborigines), and much of Africa (before its colonization by non-Africans). These racial differences in skin color are due to the size and number of the organelles in the cell that house the melanin and their distribution, as well as the shape and size of the melanin molecules. To a lesser degree, sunlight can cause skin color to darken, especially if the skin is tan or darker to begin with. But those who are like Scandinavians with very light skin color more often get sunburn and do not tan much.

Albinos who lack melanin are very vulnerable to sunburn. If they lack melanin in the inner layers of their eyes, they find glaring sunlight painful and often wear sunglasses to protect their eyes. Having melanin in your skin is important to prevent the sun's ultraviolet rays from entering your DNA in the surface skin cells and damaging those chromosomes. Sunburn is similar to the damage done by X-rays in excess doses. The major differences are in the penetration of X-rays, which go right through the body, and ultraviolet radiation, which gets no deeper than the outer layers of the skin. In addition, ultraviolet radiation produces its damage to DNA in a somewhat different way than X-rays, but the consequences are the same—they result in gene mutations or chromosome breakage leading to cell death.

This might raise a question in your mind. If melanin is so good in preventing skin cancers like melanomas and infections from blistering skin, why aren't all humans dark-skinned? The shift from dark to light skin occurred when humans moved out of Africa and across Asia and Europe. The farther north they went, the less ultraviolet radiation there was. Ultraviolet radiation is needed to make vitamin D, a process that takes place in our skin. Vitamin D is uncommon in foods outside of coastal regions where it is abundant in fish. Ultraviolet radiation is in short supply in the winter in northern latitudes. But people who live far from fish diets may become vitamin D deficient in the winter, and if they do not have sufficient vitamin D, as children get older, their bones do not grow and they become bow-legged and stunted in size. This can be a disability in a culture dependent on hunting and scavenging and traveling good distances to obtain food.

What biology, or in this case, genetics, teaches us, is that the functioning of genes has consequences. Some genes are expressed in a life cycle at a particular time and other genes are turned on (or permanently off) from fertilization to death. Some genes act when an environment triggers them to act. Cells and organisms are dynamic and there is some sort of interplay of environment and genes for many traits.

A child who is an albino is usually the product of two parents who have normal pigmentation of their skin and hair. The two parents are unaware that they are both carriers of a mutant gene that cannot make tyrosinase. When a sperm with that mutant encounters an egg with that mutant, the child will be an albino. The chance that this will happen, if both parents are carriers, is one in four. This means that of four possible encounters of the sperm and eggs, three of the children will be normal and one will be an albino. The same 3-to-1 ratio applies each time the parents succeed in getting a pregnancy.

A mutant condition that is expressed in a 3-to-1 ratio is called a recessive mutation. In the carrier, there is no obvious change in appearance. The enzymatic activity of one dose of the normal gene is sufficient to give a parent normal pigmentation no matter how dark the hair or skin color. There are about 5000 known recessive genes like this known for humans. Most of them are not nice because recessive mutations are usually the loss of a normal function, and most normal functions help us live and function successfully if we get to be born.

Single-gene Defects Come in Three Forms

Traits that involve the activities of a single pair of genes are called monogenic. The most common variety is what we have just described in the example of albinism—a rare coming into being of a child whose parents are both normal in appearance and where the odds of this happening again for those parents are one in four. Such a mutation is known as being recessive. The normal counterpart of that gene in the normal parent is given the name dominant. In general, all losses of an enzymatic function are recessive. Our metabolism involves thousands of enzymatic processes that digest molecules or synthesize molecules, and when these go wrong, some bad outcome is likely in the child. We introduce some technical terms to make sense of the status of the genes in the parents and the children. A genetic counselor would point out that the parents are both carriers or "heterozygous" for the albino trait. She would describe the albino child as being "homozygous recessive" for that trait. Children who do not get the recessive form of the gene at all are called homozygous for the dominant (in this case normal) gene.

It is not uncommon for people's eyes to glaze over reading about such technology-saturated terms. This is understandable. The world of recessive mutations striking misery into a family is relatively remote. But when it hits your family, it is quite amazing how astute your senses become to absorb information. I have seen blue-collar parents who have no more than high school educations listening and understanding far more complex explanations (often accompanied by diagrams) of their child's genetic or chromosomal condition and the likelihood of this happening again. When we are motivated, we know the lyrics of hundreds of songs, quote passages of poetry, rattle off dates of historical events, know the batting averages of every player on our favorite team, or quote chapter and verse for our favorite biblical passages. Scientists are highly motivated to know their field. But very few of those who are not scientists know or care about the science that saturates our understanding of the most fundamental issues affecting our lives.

A second category of single-gene traits involves gene mutations that are expressed in the carrier or heterozygote. Such mutations are called dominant mutations. A child born with achondroplastic dwarfism is such an example. Most people have seen them in movies like the *Wizard of Oz* (as some of the Munchkins). They have short arms and legs and a somewhat abnormal skull shape, but their torsos and heads are of normal size. In general, these are not mutations leading to a defective enzyme. They are usually mutations in a category of genes that turn on or off other genes in the developing embryo or in some organ system later in life. An example that is fairly well known of a late-onset dominant disorder is Huntington's disease. Individuals with this condition develop a progressive paralysis and loss of mental functions, usually over a period of 10–20 years. The first symptoms are most often expressed in individuals who are in their 30s.

A third group of single-gene traits involves mutant genes (usually recessive) that express in sons but not in daughters. They are called X-linked traits. They were discovered first in fruit flies in 1910 and then quickly applied to human traits such as red-green eye color deficiency (color blindness) and hemophilia. They express in sons because the genes involved for this condition are on the X chromosome. Humans have 46 chromosomes consisting of two sex chromosomes, XY in males and XX in females. The other 44 chromosomes are called autosomes because they are alike in males and females. The human X chromosome has a few thousand genes that determine a variety of traits affecting almost every organ system. The X also contains a number of genes associated with sex determination. The Y chromosome is very small and has very few genes, most of them associated with male sex determination and genes that enter into the process of forming sperm. The

Y is not necessary for life (females do not have a Y). The X is necessary for life because so many genes for vital organs are located on the X chromosome.

From this information, geneticists have classified single-gene traits as being autosomal recessive or autosomal dominant (those that follow Mendel's first law) or as being X-linked recessive (traits that are usually seen in half the sons but not the daughters of a mother who carries that mutant gene). One feature of autosomal dominant traits in humans is that usually it involves a parent who carries the dominant gene in heterozygous form with a spouse who has two of the normal gene. This puts half their future offspring at risk for getting the autosomal dominant trait like Huntington's disease.

Mendel's Second Law Describes More Complex Traits

Mendel also described a second law. He found that if two different traits, such as the color of peas and the shape of peas, are followed, a complex ratio results among the offspring of parents who are carriers for both traits. The ratio is 9:3:3:1. This is Mendel's second law. Those with both of the normal traits form 9/16 of the offspring; those with one of the normal traits expressed form 3/16; those with the other normal trait form 3/16; and those with neither normal trait form 1/16. In experiments with plants where hundreds of progeny can be obtained from crosses that yield abundant seeds, it is easy to demonstrate this law. In mammals, you need a lot of mice to produce enough offspring (several dozen) to be satisfied that it is an example of Mendel's second law. In humans, it is very difficult to demonstrate for numerous reasons. First, we rarely produce more than three or four children per family. Second, we have to find two different disorders or diseases present in the two family lines. Most of these genetic disorders are relatively uncommon so it is hard to find families like this to study. But even with these limitations, pedigrees of such rare families can be pooled and the 9:3:3:1 ratio can be shown to be operative in humans.

Human Skin Color Involves Mendel's Second Law

Although the study of individuals with two different genetic disorders is exotic at best, there are some traits that involve the activities of two or more genes to express a range of expression. Human skin color is one example. There are two major genes involved in human melanin formation and distribution in normally pigmented individuals. Instead of having a simple dominance, the trait is additive, and thus, this form of inheritance is called quantitative inheritance. Thus, most individuals from Western Africa who are dark-skinned have a genetic composition symbolized as AA BB (four genes each producing a lot of melanin). Most people of Scandinavian heritage have a skin color whose genes are represented as aa bb (four genes each producing very little melanin). If a person who is of West African composition AA BB has a spouse who is of Scandinavian composition aa bb, their off-spring will be heterozygous for both genes or Aa Bb (only two of their four genes produce a lot of melanin). Their skin color will be brown, a color intermediate between the almost black skin color in West Africa and the pale pink skin color of Scandinavians. If two such brown-skinned individuals who are products of such a racial mixture should decide to have children, they would be distributed according to Mendel's second law but with a different ratio because there is no dominance for these traits, only additivity. For the offspring of the two brown parents, 1/16 will have all four of the heavy melanin-producing genes and will be black; 4/16 will have three of the dark-determining factors and look dark brown; 6/16 will have two of the dark color factors and appear brown; 4/16 will have only one of the dark factors and look light brown; and 1/16 will be as light in skin color as a Scandinavian. This explains why some of the children of two brown-skinned parents may be darker than either parent or lighter than either parent. Of course, in such offspring, the traits for hair shape, hair color, eye color, and facial features also sort themselves out independently of the skin color genes. For this reason, Mendel's second law is called inde-pendent assortment. It arises because the genes carried by these chro-mosomes are randomly aligned with respect to each other during that cell division, meiosis, which produces sperm or eggs. The process is very much like shuffling a deck of cards.

Of importance to us as citizens is how this biology relates to racism. The heredity invoked about race is usually a set of biases passed down over the generations and circulated among slave owners justifying their bad habits of owning slaves. Racism is an aftermath of that legacy. It is also an aftermath of colonialism, where people of darker skin colors were frequently seen by their lighter skin occupiers as possessing an inferior biology. Such rationalizations work in deciding not to provide schools and job opportunities for those at the receiving end of prejudice. Note the neutrality of genetic terminology as it describes the biology of skin color formation and distribution. They differ from terms such as mulatto, quadroon, and octoroon, and similar "slave master terms," which are laden with cultural associations. They belong to an era when skin color was related to social status in an imposed "pigmentocracy." Such systems were introduced into Latin America in the 1500s but broke down in the 1600s when the three-way miscegenation of white, black, and Native American people and their assorted mixtures became more numerous and more difficult to classify. Over the centuries, such free commingling of genes leads to a diverse population with lots of blended features and a tawny skin color as the most common variety for those who are descendants of the original white colonizers.

The genetics of humans is a powerful tool for studying and often rejecting the claims of racists or those who are not exploring carefully the way the science was done about human differences. But genetics is also invoked by racists, often with sloppy standards of science, to justify their claims about the superiority of themselves or the inferiority of others. It had a role in the largely failed and largely discredited eugenics movements of the twentieth century. Learning to spot flawed scientific claims is not easy for voters or even legislators. At one time, the eugenics movement in the United States was enthusiastically supported from the President of the United States down to most columnists in respected newspapers. We should not forget, either, that the Supreme Court, in 1927, upheld the right of the state of Virginia to carry out compulsory sterilizations on Carrie Buck and her daughter, by an 8-1 vote. The evidence used in court was flawed scientifically, but because the United States was virtually completely on automatic pilot with respect to knowledge of genetics, the results were not challenged on those grounds in either the lower courts or the Supreme Court. When nine judges who were scientific illiterates can make a judgment about the validity of a claim about inheritance that was dubious to many scientists, it suggests either a failure of the judicial system in how it obtained its information or a failure of scientists with better knowledge to speak out on those issues and educate the public.

There Is a Molecular Basis of Life

The idea that molecules were associated with living things was not a surprise to chemists. But chemists, like other scientists in the early 1800s, believed that molecules associated with living organisms could not be synthesized by scientists. This turned out to be false, and urea was the first animal product that was synthesized by chemists, opening up a branch of chemistry called organic chemistry. Very quickly, chemists established that much of the material found in organisms is composed of carbon, oxygen, hydrogen, nitrogen, sulfur, and phosphorous. There were traces of other elements such as iron, sodium, potassium, chlorine, and iodine.

By the end of the nineteenth century, three major categories of organic compounds were identified. One group was the carbohydrates, which were found mostly in plants and were composed of different kinds of sugars. Starch and indigestible cellulose are carbohydrates. Chemists had less luck on the structure of proteins, the second category, which were found in abundance in meat of all kinds. They were composed of a number of smaller molecules called amino acids. Chemists had no way of synthesizing proteins or knowing how the amino acids were organized in protein molecules. They did know from studies involving the immune system, which was being studied in the late nineteenth century, that they were very numerous and virtually every protein isolated could provoke an animal such as a rabbit or a horse to produce antibodies against it. These Y-shaped antibody proteins were very specific and reacted only with the protein that provoked its formation— for example, proteins on the surface of invading bacteria.

The third category was found in two unusual sources in abundance. One was pus cells (and hence, these were mostly white blood cells) and the second was in sperm. These substances were very acidic and seemed to be present in cells with less cytoplasm and more of a nuclear presence. For that reason, this third category was called nucleic acids. In the early twentieth century, they were analyzed and shown to consist of compounds called nucleotides. Two types of nucleic acids were noted. One form had a sugar called ribose and thus the name ribonucleic acid (RNA) was assigned to it. The other category had a sugar called deoxyribose and thus those molecules were assigned the name deoxyribonucleic acid (DNA).

I realized in the mid 1980s that molecular biology was entering popular culture while I was reading and my teenage son was playing a record and I heard the phrase "Hey, hey, hey, hey! It's the DNA that makes you that way." I thought, even if I disagreed with the message (it was alluding to our behavior), I should appreciate that the molecular basis of heredity was being absorbed into rock music. Despite that entry into culture, most people still do not know how life works at a molecular level. Many people are also resistant to this idea because they fear that scientific reductionism is reducing life to "mere chemistry." Once again, the need to see ourselves as something above and beyond other animals also makes many people unhappy when thinking of themselves as self-aware multitudes of molecules.

Although it may be true that we are such assemblages of self-aware molecules, that no more defines our humanity than does an anatomist's description of us as a collection of tissue types or a multitude of cells. Even the anatomy fully described by dissecting a corpse does not define our humanity. That is because, properly, we are simultaneously a collection of molecules, a collection of cells, a collection of functioning organ systems, and, above all, possessing self-awareness made possible by our brains. Without thought and feeling, we would be less than human. At the same time, without the molecular, cellular, and anatomic organization and composition of our bodies, we can never be disembodied minds. We add to our sense of being human when we understand ourselves at all these levels—molecular, cellular, organismic, and psychological.

DNA Is Our Genetic Material

In 1950, the evidence became overwhelming that DNA is the chemical basis for the genes of the chromosomes in all cellular life. There was also a category of viruses (which are not cellular) that contained RNA instead of DNA as their genetic material. In 1953, the chemical and physical structure of DNA was worked out by James D. Watson and Francis H.C. Crick, who described the DNA molecule as a double helix similar in appearance to a spiral staircase. The DNA double helix was a magnificent contribution to science because the structure of the molecule predicts the biological activities associated with it. The molecule is crystalline and replicates by separating the two strands. The two strands are complementary, like a sandwich of a photographic positive and photographic negative. Each produces its complementary form producing two sandwiches. The sequence of nucleotide pairs that create this complementarity is nonrandom but does not follow any physical pattern. They are much like the usage of letters of the alphabet in a dictionary. We get a lot of words from a much smaller number of letters. In this respect, the letters of DNA (usually abbreviated as A, T, G, and C) are like a Morse code. We can send any English message, book length if we wish, with just dots and dashes and spaces. So, too, the DNA specifies proteins as its major role in transmitting information. This led to a search for a genetic code. It was worked out from 1960 to 1965.

Those years of 1950 to 1970 shifted the field of genetics and with it most of biological sciences from a classical approach to problems (where the chemistry had little or no role) to a molecular approach. Genes were not just names for the mutant expressions of traits. Genes were DNA and their sequences could be worked out and their products could be predicted from those sequences. It was like a Rosetta stone that could be used to decipher life at the chemical level.

Molecular Genetics Changes Human Genetics

The field of human genetics had its rebirth after World War II when it was purged of eugenics, a spurious application steeped in bias and sullied by its racism, class discrimination, social prejudices, and the Holocaust, where eugenics put into practice by the weight of the state led to genocide of a people. The new field of human genetics in 1946 was limited to advising people about their Mendelian risks if they had a child with a birth defect, but, other than electing not to have children, there was neither treatment for such children nor a means to prevent them if a pregnancy occurred. Several things changed that minimalism of choice. The first was the development of a technique called amniocentesis, which allowed physicians to transfuse blood while a fetus was in its womb and prevent a deadly disease involving an incompatibility of blood (especially the Rh blood incompatibilities). Some physicians reasoned that if they could introduce blood into a fetus by needle, why not extract amniotic fluid surrounding an embryo and examine that fetal blood for chemical or chromosomal abnormalities. That became possible in the late 1950s when the human chromosome number was shown to be 46 and one class of abnormal babies had 47 chromosomes. The first members of that class bearing 47 chromosomes had a condition then called mongoloid idiocy. After the 1970s, it was renamed as Down syndrome or trisomy 21. As the last name implies, chromosome 21 is present in triplicate instead of duplicate and is the source of the 47th chromosome.

Medical geneticists were also learning that many of the abnormalities producing birth defects could be analyzed at a biochemical level. The enzymes that were defective in most of these disorders could be assigned to a biochemical function. Amniotic fluid often revealed the missing or the abnormal product that was a telltale sign of an embryo on its way to an unhappy and often short life expectancy. This led to social changes that are still in conflict. A substantial portion of people (known as Pro-choice advocates) do not believe personhood resides in an embryo. They believe it is acquired from birth on and that the legal status of a person begins with a newborn child, not an embryo. Those who oppose this view (known as Right to Life advocates) claim personhood should have legal status at fertilization, as a zygote. There are inconsistencies on both sides to this debate. For example, if personhood begins with fertilization, shouldn't a woman who has a spontaneous miscarriage claim that aborted fetus as a dependent on her income tax for that year? Most spontaneous abortions occur very early and may be represented, if at all, by a skipped period. Should women with a skipped period in their reproductive years claim these as dependents for tax exemption? Should a woman with a miscarriage save the remains and have a full funeral for it because this was a person in the legal sense? Should such spontaneous abortions be given death certificates and a name?

For the Pro-choice advocates, there is the difficulty of assigning status to third-trimester pregnancies. Very few people would wish to abort a 7- or 8-month-old fetus, even if it were legally possible to do so (the only morally possible situations for them would be in a desperate effort to save the life of a mother). Many Pro-choice advocates do not like to define embryos or fetuses that are unmistakably human in appearance as having personhood. That is as faith-based a judgment as Right to Life advocates who assign full humanity to early embryos that have not yet developed human features (especially those from fertilization to very early stages of organogenesis).

There are limits to science. Concepts such as personhood are not sci-entific. They are cultural. A scientist describes a zygote, a blastocyst, var-ious stages of organogenesis, fetal status when organogenesis stops, and birth when a child is delivered vaginally or surgically removed. These terms can be applied to any mammal. Think of it this way. If you break an eggshell to fry an egg sunny-side up and you note a tiny red spot near the yolk, which is evidence that it is a fertilized egg in an early stage of development, are you eating a fried egg or a fried chicken? Does the red spot confer "chickenhood" to the egg?

The ethical and moral issues will not go away through scientific findings because the former are faith-based and the latter are reason-based. Medical science has chosen diagnosis and treatment as its pre-ferred aim and diagnosis and prevention as a secondary aim of its health policy. Where treatment is not possible, prevention is the backup. But there are two issues here. Prevention in the case of infectious diseases that can kill large numbers of people allows the state to impose quaran-tines or to pass compulsory immunization laws. We sacrifice total free-dom of choice for protection of society as a whole during an epidemic or to prevent one. Some libertarians oppose this and feel that everyone should be free to make good or bad choices. But this can lead to the death of people who are not able to pay for immunizations or who are unaware they are available or who cannot hide out in a safe place until the epidemic passes. In an unequal society, you cannot have complete freedom. A major role of the government is to protect its people. The second issue involves the interpretation of prevention. We think of immunization in favorable terms because we allow our immune system to be mobilized against a microbe that we consider hazardous. But pre-vention of birth by abortion is filled with faith-based points of view. At one extreme are those who would consider it murder to prevent a fer-tilized egg from adhering to the surface of the uterine endometrium, but would they want to execute the woman who elected this procedure for birth control as premeditated murder or send her to prison for decades? At the other extreme are those who feel prevention of birth by abortion is preferable to raising a child who will require immense sacrifice, suf-fer a lot of pain, or experience a shortened life expectancy with little opportunity to experience life as normal people know it. I emphasize again that these are faith-based decisions and not scientific ones. At pre-sent, the United States has a secular government with a separation of church and state. Imposing the religious or moral values of one group of its citizens on those whose religious or moral views differ is a tension that is solved by courts or cultural consensus and not by science itself.

The use of DNA to analyze birth defects through prenatal diagnosis is an innovation that began in the late 1980s and has become a very powerful tool for genetic medicine. Even if the product produced by the gene cannot be isolated, if that gene is shown to be the cause of the disorder, it can be detected by prenatal diagnosis. Every mutation has a signature of its defect in the DNA. For some diseases, the use of prenatal diagnosis has led to a virtual disappearance of it in at-risk families. Terrible disorders involving lysosomal storage disease, disorders that disturb profoundly the ability to learn or to coordinate the body, and disorders that lead to profound disabilities are usually stopped in gestation when diagnosed. This is also true for chromosomal abnormalities that are incompatible with life after birth (such as trisomy 13 or trisomy 18) or severely limit that life (such as trisomy 21). The prevailing philosophy in the field of genetic services is that the autonomy of the prospective parents should be followed when they are given bad news about the biochemical or chromosomal prospects for their yet to be born embryo. Genetic counselors do not advocate and do not judge a client. They see their role as providing information. Physicians who do the elective abortion see their role as applying preventive medicine. There are, of course, physicians who will not perform abortions. That is a legitimate exercise of their faith-based beliefs. But just as judges excuse themselves from cases where they have a personal interest of some sort, physicians are ethically bound not to hide information if the patients ask for their options or would obtain it from other physicians. In medicine today, it is the patient who makes the decision of what option to choose, not the physician.

Molecular Genetics May Lead to Treatments of Genetic Disorders

Most physicians see themselves primarily as healers. If given the opportunity, they would prefer to see birth defects treated rather than prevented by elective abortion. The use of molecular tools to insert genes into cells may lead to "gene replacement therapy." So far, it is still largely an imagined rather than an applied field of medicine. Early tests of introducing genes also introduced tumors because the agents to carry the genes into cells were viruses thought to be benign but unexpectedly were capable of inducing cancers. Those gene therapy studies have been halted until a new delivery system can be worked out. Even then, it may turn out that randomly inserting normal genes into mutant cells may have unexpected consequences later in life. It will take years of trial-and-error procedures in animal models and human clinical trials before that method becomes routine. If it does work, most physicians will provide gene therapy as an option for pregnancies that are at risk, and many of the clients will elect this option rather than abortion, which they may look upon as a last resort option.

From a long-range perspective, there are problems with the treatment approach. Biologists see life as having an origin that may be 3 billion years in the past and they may see humans as members of our species, *Homo sapiens*, as being around for about another 1 million years in the form we know. If we patch up genetic defects that would have died before reproductive maturity or if we patch up sterile couples through in vitro fertilization and other procedures that allow the infertile to become parents with their own gametes, we act in opposition to the role of natural selection. This leads to an accumulation of genes that would have been normally eliminated. How many generations can gene therapy be applied at the somatic level (the target tissues expressing disease) before the burden of mutations in society becomes excessive? If we shift gene therapy to include reproductive cells, this would change the outcome but it would mean some sort of conscious eugenics would be applied. The history of our earlier attempts at eugenics is not very good, and society needs to go slow before embarking on ambitious plans to weed out undesirable genes. This may not be a problem if the choices are voluntary and the autonomy of the users is based on carefully weighed information and alternative options are available to them.

Human Molecular Biology Gives Us an Enriched Understanding

Health is not the only use of the knowledge of our molecular biology. From studies in the last third of the twentieth century, geneticists and biochemists have followed the evolution of molecules such as hemoglobin. The hemoglobin genes involved are on two different chromosomes.

Some of those genes are dead or nonfunctioning (called pseudogenes) and are relics of our past ancestry. We can see where they arose in the primate line or even earlier. This has been greatly enhanced by studies of the DNA in different species because genes in most living things are more complex and have more components than those parts that form the proteins themselves. By studying these sequences stuck between the informational parts, an even larger abundance of past mutations (having no harmful effect on hemoglobin or other large protein) can be studied. They can be used to trace the migration of people from the time our ancestors left Africa some 50,000 years ago to the various ethnic groups around the world.

A good example of this evolutionary history by studying present and past human genes is the study of the genes involved with color perception. There is a set of duplicate genes on the human X chromosome that produces molecules called opsins. These molecules are found in the cone cells of the retina. Cone cells see color and rod cells are the black- and white-detecting cells of the retina. There are two major opsin genes on the X chromosome; one is sensitive to wavelengths that lead a person to detect green. The other leads to the detection of red. In most instances of red-green color blindness, there is an unusual breakage and reunion of these duplicate genes leading to triplications or quadruplicating of these opsin genes. Some of these changes have no effect on color vision (if there is an intact red-seeing opsin and an intact green-seeing opsin). But if the recombined product has only one of these intact and the other is too big or too small because of the rearranged DNA, the person will be red-deficient or green-deficient. It may be mild or it may be severe. One can test people for color detection by a variety of tools. One of the most common is a set of charts showing dotted numbers against a dotted background. All four possibilities can be diagnosed—severe or mild red or green deficiency.

The person who first recognized color blindness as an inherited disorder was Joseph Dalton, the founder of the atomic theory in chemistry in 1810. He and several of his male relatives had red-green color blindness. Dalton wondered if it was caused by some discoloring of the fluid in his eyes and he willed his eyes to medicine to study them. When he died, the fluid was found to be normal and his eyeballs were placed in a vial and stored. In the 1990s, someone got the idea to do a DNA analysis of Dalton's eyes and his opsin genes were sequenced. The specific defect he had, a severe red-detecting defect, could be diagnosed. Think about that. Well over 100 years after Dalton died, the DNA of his genes was able to provide scientists with the information needed to diagnose his condition.

The opsin genes can also be traced to primates and earlier vertebrates such as fish. An ancient fish ancestor that gave rise to land animals, the coelacanth, has the opsin gene for seeing blue but not for seeing red or green. The red or green opsin genes (or both) can also be detected in various mammals, allowing biologists to identify which are likely to recognize specific colors for behavioral tests.

In 1967, I gave a public lecture at UCLA in which I was asked to speculate about the future of my field. The genetic code had been recently worked out and I thought that in a century or less we would have the tools to sequence DNA. I reasoned that if mummies could be blood-typed, this meant that their proteins survived in their desiccated tissues. If this were true for proteins, it should be true for the DNA; but DNA is a more complex molecule because it is organized in long threads that are chopped up when a person dies. However, I felt that if the fragments, when sequenced, could be compared to other fragments by computers and a matching sequence could be extended by this means, it should be possible to recreate the genotype of the dead. I gave a name to this new field, "necrogenetics," which happily did not take, but the publicity I got was worldwide. I got letters from a nurse in France whose son had committed suicide and she wondered if his DNA could be used to make a twin of him. I also got angry letters including one from a woman in McKeesport, Pennsylvania, who said "if you were my son, I would beat you with a broom handle." I also got newspaper clippings sent by former students with headlines like "King Tut May Become a Papa." About a generation later, much to my surprise and delight at its rapidity, that imagined possibility became real when the field of paleogenetics emerged and the sequences of extinct animals, such as passenger pigeons, mammoths, and quaggas, could be analyzed. For the past 10 years, the sequences of genes in Neanderthal ancestors have been accumulating, and by the end of this century, if enough ancient bones and teeth are found, a complete sequence may be available.

The applications of DNA sequencing to evolutionary biology have been enormously helpful in confirming the relations determined by classical methods and in resolving many relations that could not be decided by such means. We saw that a new field of comparative genomics exists that is a major part of evolutionary biology today. A surprise finding was the comparison of a major gene for hair color in Neanderthal DNA and human DNA. Neanderthals would have had red hair if this gene were expressed in them as in contemporary humans. I like to think of these genomes as analogous to blueprints used by engineers to plan how a large building is constructed. Several hundred such genomes have been sequenced and by the end of the twenty-first century, that number will be in the thousands or tens of thousands across all 92 of our phyla, from viruses to humans. For biologists, this will be a history of life as well as an opportunity to isolate genes associated with the formation of the nervous system to learn how neurons work in groups to store memory, to relate ideas, and to initiate activities from speech to running.

Recommended Reading

Sean B. Carroll's *The making of the fittest: DNA and the ultimate forensic record of evolution* (2006. W.W. Norton, New York) gives a superb overview of how genetics works and how it can be used at the molecular level.

CHAPTER 10

We Have a Life Cycle and Sexuality That Is Genetically Programmed

F OR MOST OF HUMANITY, FOR MOST OF THE TIME that humans have been self-aware these past 130,000 years, the human life cycle ran from birth to old age and death. There was a vaguely understood pregnancy that was interpreted as beginning somewhere just before monthly menstruation stopped; but where that beginning was—in the oviduct leading to the uterus or that it involved the union of a single sperm with a single egg— was not known until late in the nineteenth century. The next event a woman experienced (other than morning sickness) was referred to as "quickening," when the first stirrings of the fetus made its presence known in the womb. It took place anywhere from the 23rd to the 25th week of pregnancy. For many a medieval theologian, quickening was the event signaling the entry of the soul into the future baby. This made sense for a dualistic view of human life that identified a soul as animating the corpse-like body that remains when death occurs and the soul leaves.

Descriptive embryology was a product of debates in the 1700s. There were two contending views. Some believed that embryos were just enlargements of a preformed tiny baby that resided in the egg. That view came from studies of insects like aphids that show such baby aphids in the abdomens of their mothers. This argument is known as preforma- tion—the baby is preformed. One implication for some preformationists of the time was that each generation has one less miniature baby residing in the ovaries than the previous generation, and when Christ returns, the last of these generations will have been spent. Opposed to the idea of preformation was the view of a developmental process in which complexity emerged in gradual stages by unknown processes different from simple enlargement or growth. That view was known as epigenesis. It turned out to be correct when better microscopes were applied in the late 1700s to the embryos of chickens and frogs.

Experimental Embryology Tries to Explain How Development Occurs

Experimental embryology began in the 1890s with studies of the very early stages of development. After fertilization, the egg is called a zygote. The zygote begins to divide by ordinary cell division or mitosis and produces what were called blastomeres when I was a student. Today, these are called stem cells. In some species, these stem cells have a twinning capacity. An isolated cell from a two- or four-cell stage can form an identical twin of the remaining cells in sea urchins and many other animals. This is probably true for human twins that arise before the embryo leaves the oviduct and enters the uterus. Human twins formed after implantation are housed in a common membrane of a structure called a blastocyst. Such twins (about 80% of identical twins) have a collection and distribution of membranes in the placenta that make them identifiable instantly as identical twins. The other 20% of human identical twins cannot be identified by their placental membranes because they had separated into two masses of stem cells before the blastocyst structure had formed shortly after leaving the oviduct. Those 20% of identical twins have placental membranes like most people who are singletons (or twins who are not identical).

Experimental embryologists also did a number of studies to explore what initiates a pregnancy or life cycle. Some scientists learned that a sperm was not needed to get the egg to divide and form stem cells. The egg could be stimulated with the prick of a needle and the process enhanced if different chemicals were added to the eggs before stabbing them. This process is called parthenogenesis (which is Greek for virgin birth). Very few parthenogenetic eggs went on to form a normal embryo and most abort whether this is done in invertebrates or vertebrates. But some species have a natural parthenogenesis, aphids being one such class of organisms producing only daughters from their mothers. The lesson from partheno-genesis is that the sperm has two roles in initiating pregnancy: It con-tributes half the hereditary material to the nucleus of the zygote and it ini-tiates the mitotic process by mechanical stimulation of the egg.

Scientists quickly isolated three components to development: growth, differentiation, and movement. Growth is measured by the number of cell divisions that take place and an increase in mass of liv-ing matter. Differentiation involves a progressive change in function of the cells as they lose their potential to form twins and are stuck in the tissue type to which they belong. Finally, movement of cells allows groups of cells to slide together or slip under another layer or form bulges and pockets in the developing embryo. The first evidence that these processes are under genetic control came from studies of slime molds. The species *Dictyostelium discoides* is a slime mold that starts as a group of ameboid cells. They are irregularly shaped and resemble the protozoan amebas frequently seen by teenage students in their science classes. These amebas reach a critical mass and then begin streaming toward a center, and as the cells come in contact, they adhere to one another and form a slug-like organism that begins to slide on a secreted lubricant (hence, the term slime molds). As the slug moves forward, it begins to lift one end and thin out a tall stalk on which a globular spore chamber forms. The object looks like a tiny plant of some sort (and its cell walls are rich in cellulose-like plant carbohydrates). The spore case bursts and the released spores hatch out a new generation of amebas.

Studies of these slime molds showed that some mutations arose that prevented streaming. Other mutations allowed slug formation but no differentiation into the stalked form. There were some mutations that led to bush-like multiple-stalked adult forms. The difficulty with slime molds was that they did not have a known sex life. There was no way to get these different forms to mate with each other to do the sort of breed-ing that geneticists love to do in order to map genes and combine them in different ways to study their effects.

A different approach that was genetic was initiated by Edward B. Lewis. He used fruit flies and studied a number of mutant forms of a gene called *bithorax*. Some of these genes controlled the formation of body segments and determined if they would form wing, balancer, leg, or abdominal segment appearance in their adult form. He combined many of these gene mutations and produced four-winged flies (fruit flies have two wings) or flies with half-wing formation, or eight-legged flies instead of six-legged flies. He discovered a class of gene mutations that determined the developmental fate of the body segments of insects. Lewis's work was important in our understanding of how evolution occurred in the arthropods (organisms such as lobsters, millipedes, insects, and spiders). It gave molecular biologists an opportunity to identify the way developmental genes worked.

You can think of an insect as a set of boxes. Genes are turned on in different boxes in response to chemical signals (usually a gradient from high dose to low dose of the signal). In response to the signal, one pair of boxes near the head region may produce antennae, another pair of boxes may produce eyes, another pair of boxes may produce mouth parts for grasping food, another pair of boxes farther down the sequence of boxes may produce forelegs, and still farther, a pair of boxes may produces mid-body legs; this may be followed by formation of wings and so on down to the tail end of the train of box pairs.

What is amazing to contemplate is that these developmental genes that lead to differentiation of segments (called *Hox* genes) are found in us. We do not think of ourselves as segmented, but if we look at a mammal's early embryonic body, we would see the segmentation (called somites) of the mammalian body from head to tail.

Some Implications of the Human Life Cycle

We have about 25,000 genes. Each is represented twice in the nucleus of a zygote. From those genes, instructions are first poured out to set up the processes of growth, differentiation, and morphogenetic movements. The embryo differentiates accordingly, forming three major tissues that form three tube-like layers. The outermost layer will give rise to the skin and the nervous system. The innermost layer or tube will give rise to the digestive tract along with the lungs, liver, and pancreas. The middle layer will form the muscles, circulatory system, kidneys, bones, and bulk of body padding that we call connective tissue. Each of these embryonic tissues involves the activities of hundreds of genes guiding them into the rudiments seen in the early embryo. Each specific organ derived from these tissues also requires hundreds or thousands of genes. We can imagine the developmental process much like a symphony orchestra, with the interplay of the different batches of genes much like the conductor's use of strings, woodwinds, brass, or percussion to bring about a harmonious event in our minds that fills us with aesthetic pleasure. So, too, life presents this grand symphony at a molecular and cellular level as we gradually emerge from the activities of the genes of that first zygotic nucleus.

The dark side of our contemplation is that genes mutate, and some of these mutant genes may disturb the developmental process and lead to birth defects. Some will lead to apparently normal-looking organ systems that do not quite work as well as normal ones and may shorten our life expectancy. Still others may be the lucky recipients of genes that give more than normal efficiency and lead to athletic records among those who are fortunate to harbor them. If a group of genes gives us better memories or better relating of things, or gives us that hard-to-define quality we call creativity, it can lead to a potential for eminence. You can have athletic potential from your genes but not be interested in sports. You can have perfect pitch and a musical memory but lack an interest or an opportunity to cultivate a career in music. You may be a creative genius, but your culture gives you no opportunity to earn a living except as an unskilled laborer. Life is more complex than the outcomes of our genes, but it is dependent on those genes for whatever talents we try to cultivate.

The knowledge of the biology of our life cycle also gives us insights into how genes act later in our lives. Are we just let go after reaching 18 or so years with no further gene activity leading to change? That is not likely. There are genes that govern cell death, and as we age, more of our cells self-destruct in response to those genes. We know there are genes that lead to premature aging syndromes like progeria, with children of 8 or 10 years looking like senescent adults in their 80s and dying before they reach their adult years. We know from studies of identical twins that they continue to look alike in middle age as well as old age, even if they are raised apart.

We also know that the properties that govern normal cell interactions can be disturbed and lead to tumor cell formation. There may be dozens of genes involved in tumor cell formation. Normal cells in a tissue have an adhesiveness that holds them together. We do not have muscle cells from our arms or legs migrating into our blood vessels and lodging into our brains to form a muscular tumor. Many properties have to change besides loss of adhesiveness for a metastatic (spreading) tumor to emerge. The normal cells also have a regulated cell division that turns them off for long periods of time when they are acting as adult tissues.

Tumor cells have one or more mutations that lead to uncontrolled cell division and these cells heap up in mounds and crowd normal tissue. The resumption of cell division in adult tissues where almost all of the cells are nondividing is also regulated by gene mutations of the cell cycle. There are several dozen genes involved in mitosis that keep it orderly and in tune with the rest of the cells of a tissue. This makes cancer a genetic disease not in the sense that we inherit cancers (only a few are inherited) but in the sense that tumors in the body arise in tissues such as bone, liver, gut, lung, breast, prostate, or brain from changes in normal genes. These are accidents of living and not passed on to our offspring.

Some gene sequences make a person more prone to cancers, that is, they increase their risk. One well-known example is the gene *BRCA* in women, which raises their likelihood of developing breast cancer. Factors in their diet may be involved; exposure to chemical agents or radiations may be involved. A cell without this gene could require a half dozen or so independent mutations at the right genes to convert it into a tumor cell, whereas a cell carrying the *BRCA* gene may only need one or two such hits to trigger tumor cell formation.

Although it may make nonscientists frightened to think of all the things that can go wrong in a human life cycle, it is also of immense importance for each of us to know this information because we can reduce our risks. Knowledge of how cells work, how genes work, what causes mutations, what agents we are exposed to, and how we can lessen that exposure are very important to having healthier lives. Think of it this way. You know you could be killed by a psychotic person as a random act of violence. You could also be killed in a war you did not help create and whose reason for being you do not like but out of duty you nevertheless will serve. You could be killed if your car crashes, if your plane crashes, or if your boat sinks. You could fall off a ladder, choke on a hunk of beef jammed into your trachea, or slip on a hardwood floor and crack your skull. You could burn to death trapped in your bedroom. The list of hazards is endless. We know all this, but it does not prevent us from living. Most of us practice what I call "defensive living," and we reduce our risks where we can, knowing that there is always an uncertainty to our lives. I am just adding one more level of uncertainty, one that is more likely to kill you or your children than any of the rare events I described. Why not open our culture to knowledge of science and practice defensive living at the genetic level?

Chromosomes, Genes, and Hormones
Determine Our Sexuality

Sex is controversial because we move back and forth among three levels of knowledge. The first is biological. Males are usually XY and females are usually XX in their sex chromosome composition, which means that our biological sex is set at fertilization. The genitalia of males and females differ and that difference is biologically determined. The second level occurs after birth and involves both hormonal changes in our teen years and an abundant amount of cultural influences that tell us what is expected of most males and most females in a particular society. The third level is more difficult to assign. It involves behaviors that are claimed to be innate because of alleged exposure to hormones while still in utero that lead to a set of male behaviors or a set of female behaviors. The evidence for this is much less compelling than for the first two levels of our understanding. This third level is also the one most subject to rationalizations for improper behavior, gender discrimination, infidelity, sex role confusion, sex orientation confusion, bullying, and other manifestations of alleged innate aggression (male-associated) or innate sensitivity to others (female-associated). It is this third level that is invoked whenever evolutionary psychology tries to account for the alleged origins of human sexual behavior. Because most people are only acquainted with the second level (which they have experienced), they are likely to confuse biological claims that are spurious or unproven with biological events that are real but which are not known to humanity save for a sprinkling of biologists and physicians who have studied sex determination as a developmental process.

Sex is also controversial because it is one of the most charged psychological experiences humans have. Courtship, marriage, child-rearing, rape, homosexuality, premarital sex, masturbation, prostitution, birth control, abortion, and sex prejudice are very much part of most human experience since antiquity. One of the roles of religion has been to carefully define what males and females can do, when and with whom, and with proper sanctioning of society usually through its religious traditions and theology.

I used to teach my students that there are seven sexes of humans. Five of these belong to the first level and are highly determined by biology. One is very much associated with our second level of understanding sex. The seventh is associated with our third level of understanding.

The seven sexes I call our chromosomal sex, gonadal sex, internal genital sex, external genital sex, our genetic sex, our pubertal sex, and our cultural, legal, or psychological sex. To understand our sexual biology, we need to know some of the embryonic players in this process. Every human embryo about the time it is 6 weeks old has a pair of structures called the gonads. These are the future reproductive structures called ovaries in females and testes in males. Every embryo about this same time forms two tubular or ductal structures that are near these gonads. These are called the Wolffian and the Mullerian ducts. They are involved in the future internal genitalia of males and females. In addition, every embryo by its tenth week of existence develops an external set of genital rudiments. These rudiments will eventually form the penis and scrotum in males and vaginal pudenda (labia and clitoris) in females.

How Our Sex Is Determined in the First 60 Days of Pregnancy

Chromosomal sex is determined at fertilization and it is the sperm that determines whether a zygote will be male (from a Y-chromosome-bearing sperm) or female (from an X-chromosome-bearing sperm). Eggs normally contribute a single X to their offspring. The Y chromosome contains a gene for shifting the gonad from a neutral condition to a testis. It does so through a gene on the Y called *SRY*. If that *SRY* gene is normal, it will do its job. In the absence of *SRY*, the neutral gonad differentiates into an ovary. How do we know this?

In the XX neutral gonad, the primordial germ cells that are XX enter the outer layer of the neutral gonad. The cells spread themselves along this outer layer and become the ovarian epithelium that will eventually form the blister-like follicles that produce the eggs each month in a woman's reproductive years. In an XX normal embryo, the gonads do not produce these two hormones. The absence of the nonsteroid hormone allows the Mullerian ducts to form the oviducts and uterus and upper vagina. The absence of testosterone leads to self-destruction of the Wolffian ducts. In a sense, the female development is the default or normal tendency of differentiation of the embryonic rudiments because if you use a mammal like a rabbit or rat, you can remove the neutral gonads in an XY embryo and instead of a male rabbit or male rat, you will get a female with internal uterus, oviducts, and vagina.

The external genitalia are the last of the organ systems involving reproduction to be produced. At about the 55th day of pregnancy, both XX and XY embryos produce three embryonic rudiments where the belly and legs meet. They are called the genital folds, the genital swellings, and the genital tubercle. In response to a testosterone hormone produced by the embryonic testes of the XY normal human embryo, the genital folds enlarge, elongate, and form a tubular structure, the penile shaft. At the far end of this shaft is the genital tubercle that forms the head of the penis. The genital swellings enlarge and move in the opposite direction to the penile shaft and swoop around to form a sac, called the scrotum. Later, in the third term of pregnancy, the testes will descend from the abdomen into the scrotum.

In the female, the absence of that testosterone hormone causes the genital folds to form the labia minora, the genital swellings form the labia majora, and the genital tubercle becomes the clitoris. Note that in the formation of the female external genitals, it is the absence of the testosterone that is involved. How do we know this? Because in rabbits or rats, you can remove the testes of the XY embryo before the genital folds, swellings, and tubercle have differentiated and they will form the female pudenda.

Abnormal Anatomic Sexual Development
Is Frequently Chromosomal or Genetic

Some babies are born with ambiguous genitals. One category is called hermaphroditic and the second is called pseudohermaphroditic. Hermaphrodites have both male and female gonadal components. What does this mean? They may have one ovary and one testis or they may have two ovotestes. There are many other permutations but they all indicate contradictory male and female hormones in the adult and some confusion about how the embryo will form the internal and external genitalia. There are several mechanisms that can bring this about. One of these is cellular chimerism. Babies with this condition have XY cells and XX cells. How on earth does that happen? In nonidentical twins, half of them are a boy and half are a girl, produced by two eggs, one fertilized by a Y-bearing sperm and the other fertilized by an X-bearing sperm. Imagine if the two fertilized eggs, instead of forming twins, are stuck together and form a singleton. That singleton is the chimera. What should have been a boy twin and a girl twin is one individual with two different genetic constitutions populating its cells.

Pseudohermaphrodites are babies that have a contradiction between their gonads and their external genitals. The baby might have ovaries, but at birth, the attending physician sees a penis and scrotum. Sometimes the scrotum is incompletely closed, and if the physician probes the opening, it may reveal a vaginal channel and a uterus. If the pseudohermaphrodite has ovaries, it is called a female pseudohermaphrodite. If the baby is born with female genitalia present but testes are present inside the body cavity, that baby will be raised as a female and may not know of the presence of testes until her teen years when she fails to menstruate and a medical examination reveals those internal testes. Such a pseudohermaphrodite is called a male pseudohermaphrodite. Dozens of types of pseudohermaphrodites are known. Some involve failures of the steroid hormone pathway and abnormal amounts of male hormone flood the developing female embryo. Sometimes it is the absence of testosterone in an XY embryo that leads to a male pseudohermaphrodite. The conditions can vary in severity in complications and some can be life-threatening. The steroid pathway defects sometimes lead to an inability to maintain salt in the cells.

There are probably hundreds of genes involved in the production of the human reproductive system. Putting it together requires that the sex chromosome number be normal and that the genes involved be normal. When nature's errors are present, abnormalities result. If we are biologically ignorant, we just think in terms of a disease or abnormality requiring medical attention. If we are biologically literate, we can think of life as a remarkable process involving the participation of thousands of genes throughout our life cycle turning on and turning off, coordinated by those signals that cells release and respond to. The knowledge won by scientific studies allows us to predict what consequences will occur if a hormone is not produced, or if a receptor for that hormone no longer recognizes it, or if genes are shifted from one chromosome to another. Instead of bizarre oddities and surprises, we have an understanding of what went wrong; in some cases, there are medical remedies, and in some cases, there are no medical solutions to the difficult life some children and their parents will have to experience. Science may provide understanding and it may lead to effective treatment, but science is not magic and not all problems afflicting a baby can be solved by science.

Psychological Sex Provides the Most Controversy

Do we have a psychological sex? Some people prefer to think of all behavior as acquired or cultural and thus they do not accept claims that males and females show differences in behavior either in response to hormones or in what are called innate gender roles. Others think that many sex differences are innate and are wired into our brains by the presence or absence of testosterone or the presence or absence of estrogens at critical times in the formation of our brains. Still others believe that there are genes which determine if we are male-oriented or female-oriented, resulting in heterosexual attraction or homosexual attraction. Many believe that there are evolutionary (and hence genetically programmed) reasons why males and females differ in their behavior in most cultures. There is evidence on both sides of the debate, and it is not easy to give an answer that satisfies skeptics or adherents regarding any of these issues.

In female pseudohermaphrodites, most of these XX individuals, whether raised as males or raised as females (and if raised as females, whether or not they had surgery in infancy to remove the penis and scrotum), identify themselves as thinking, feeling, and acting as males more than females. Male pseudohermaphrodites who are XY but who are identified as females from birth (because they have a vagina and female pudenda) have a female identity throughout their lives. They have internal testes but they lack receptors to the testosterone they produce. The difficulty with these studies is that the conditions are rare. Skeptics like to be overwhelmed, but if they are wedded to an ideological view, even being overwhelmed rarely shakes their faith. This is as true for those who favor a biological determinism of sexual behavior as for those who reject it.

Compounding the difficulty in assessing these studies is that some of the people who are drawn to the field have their own biases and may unconsciously let their scientific guard down and publish poorly controlled studies. Many of the initial claims that there is a gene for male homosexuality have not been confirmed by other studies done independently by other investigators. Unless fraud is involved (and it rarely is), such flawed papers just stop being cited but they are not retracted.

We do not like to hear scientists say "the jury is still out" or "I don't know." We like answers and not wishy-washy statements about things that matter to us. Once again, this has a lot to do with the way the public learns science—often in sensational presentations in the mass media and in dull and uninspiring ways in the classroom. Honest discussion and debate are rare. Critical reflection is replaced by synthetic opposition or overstated claims. Admitting that science does not know is interpreted as a defect of science.

There are very few controlled large-scale experiments done on humans involving invasive or physiological changes. It is immoral to do experiments on that scale even if those persons give consent. One exception was a study during World War II on homosexual soldiers. It was thought that giving testosterone to them would shift them to heterosexual behavior. It did not. As is often the case in human studies, animal studies are substituted for the basis of our claims. This may not be wrong; it just does not dent the skepticism of those with a cultural interpretation of all human behavior. When XX mice embryos are stressed with testosterone in utero, after their sexual development has led to formation of female genitalia, those mice, as adults, show intercourse mounting behavior as if they are males.

Gender studies involve multiple human activities. Let us sort out some of these. The ones most likely to be associated with innate factors are those involved in courtship attraction. We are not taught to fall in love with someone else. It happens, and why we are attracted to some people and not to others of our peers is not known. But about 2–3% of males will be attracted to other males. The same is true for females. Studies by sexologists like Alfred Kinsey identified an even larger percent of males or females who had some homosexual experience or feelings but who identified themselves as heterosexual.

A second class of gender studies involves attitudes of sex-identity. Males think of themselves as male and females think of themselves as female. They look upon the behavior of the other sex as showing different behaviors from their own. This might be attitudes toward crying during times of emotional stress. It might be for play preferences as children (teachers and parents often remark that little boys tend to be more energized in their play than little girls). The problem with such differences, which are real, is that they could be products of cultural training and picked up from the modeling or mimicry that establishes so much of our social behavior.

The least likely innate gender differences are activities involving academic success, occupation, creativity, leadership, and other qualities associated with status and earning a living. In only one generation since the sexual revolutions of the 1980s, women have become powerful politicians, Supreme Court judges, CEOs of corporations, Nobel laureates, TV news anchors, the majority of medical students, and where barriers have been relaxed, fully capable of competing with men for top positions and honors.

If there are genetic programs for male or female behavior triggered by hormonal exposure in utero, these will emerge as the human genome is teased apart into the functions of our 25,000 genes, at least 6000 of which are associated with our nervous system. I suspect that our answers will emerge from these molecular approaches, rather than from the more speculative approaches associated with "black box" psychological studies or inferred evolutionary adaptations to past environments.

Recommended Reading

Sean Carroll is a leading advocate of "evo-devo," a developmental biology approach to how we emerge from fertilized egg to newborn baby and how that is connected to evolution. His book, *Endless forms most beautiful: The new science of evo devo and the making of the animal kingdom* (2005. Norton, New York), is well worth reading.

For a more detailed account of "the seven sexes of man," see my text, *Human genetics.* Chapter 19. Sex determination: The seven levels of human sexuality, pp. 268–282 (1984. D.C. Heath, Lexington, Massachusetts).

CHAPTER 11

Neurobiology Reveals How the Brain Works

UNTIL THE SEVENTEENTH CENTURY, the brain was thought to be a place where the blood was cooled. We still use the popular phrase "hot-blooded" to refer to people with a temper. When diarist Samuel Pepys in 1664 described a young man about to receive a transfusion of blood from a sheep, he noted that he was being treated to cool his brain because of the madness noted by his colleagues. The idea that the brain itself was the source of our self-awareness was developed much later and not without a great deal of false leads, such as phrenology, which tried to interpret personality and talents by bumps on the skull presumably produced by the corresponding brain mass that existed beneath them.

There are four ways we have learned about what we call the mind. The oldest comes from studies by theologians and philosophers. Theirs can be called an inferential approach based on observations of individual and group behavior. That approach gave us concepts like the soul, original sin, possession by the devil or his agents, ghosts, extrasensory perception, and revelation. It also generated models of human nature that were often contradictory. None of these can merit the designation of being scientific. The field of psychology, which developed in the nineteenth century, especially in Germany, England, and France, gave us more insights about behavior and how it could be measured and studied through experimentation. Francis Galton's laboratory in the last half of the nineteenth century was a major source of insights (not all correct) about human behavior and human abilities, including human intelligence. He was also the first to suggest using twin studies. The field of psychiatry used a different approach by inferring normal mental functions from neurotic or psychopathic individuals. We associate Sigmund Freud with his great insights into the conflicts that led to aberrant behavior and his attempt to use "talk therapy" to bring those conflicts to self-awareness in the patient. The fourth of these approaches we call neurobiology. It involves studies of brain function through injuries to specific areas of the brain, genetic disorders of the brain, studies of neuron function, and instrumentation, such as NMR (nuclear magnetic resonance) and PET (positron emission tomography), to identify areas of the brain that "light up" when the subject is asked to perform certain activities. Note that psychology, psychiatry, and neurobiology are all valid scientific attempts to understand how the brain works.

Psychology has traditionally used what some call a "black box" approach. Stimuli go into the brain and behavior (responses) comes out. From controlled experiments using test subjects, quite a lot about behavior was learned, but virtually nothing was learned about where this occurs in the brain and how the brain works at a cellular or physiological level. Psychiatry before the 1960s was almost entirely a field of "talk therapy," the best known of which was Freud's own psychoanalytic techniques. Most scientists today do not see Freud's approach as revealing much about how the brain works because it is similar to psychology in using a black box approach. What Freud did recognize is that we engage in activities like repression and sublimation that were not studied by nineteenth-century psychology. Freud alerted us to a dynamic process going on in our brains that could spill over into antisocial behavior or self-defeating behavior. In the last half of the twentieth century, surgical studies, physiological studies, and pharmaceutical studies have shown there were treatments that were more effective in treating pathological conditions that did not respond to talk therapy.

Neurobiology studies the brain itself. Our brain contains about 100 billion neurons. The brain is very convoluted, but if its surface were all flattened out, the brain would be similar in size to a tablecloth that could accommodate a table for four diners. The fundamental unit of the brain is the neuron and the fundamental unit of the neuron is the synapse. A synapse is a connection of fibers produced by elongated extensions of neurons called axons and a bushy growth of fibers at their ends collectively called dendrites. Neurobiologists have learned how nerve pulses are transmitted. Calcium ions play a major role. At the synaptic junctions between one of the fibers from a transmitting neuron to a fiber in a receiving neuron, there are chemicals (known as neurotransmitters) present both in the synaptic fibers and in the surrounding space around them that permit the nerve impulse to move from neuron to neuron. A single neuron may have hundreds, even thousands, of fiber extensions to other neurons. Networks are the major way information flows through the brain.

The Synapse as the Basis of Brain Function

A major insight into brain function was made by Donald Hebb in 1949. He noted that neurons that are "wired" together by a synapse will fire together, and the more they are activated, the more permanent the association of the synapse becomes. Studies of synapse formation show that neurons produce new synaptic fibers at a fixed rate and occasionally fibers from different neurons join together. If there is no reinforcement by firing activity, these associations decay and new fibers are formed and make new associations. If a particular connection or network performs a useful function, Hebb's law comes into play: "Synapses that fire together stay together."

A good example of how neurobiology clarifies mental phenomena can be seen in the analysis of the phantom limb phenomenon. A person who loses an arm may feel the amputated limb as if it were actually there, and experience touch and pain. As the weeks pass by, the phantom limb seems to shrink and eventually it may feel as if it is only a hand that is stroking one's cheek. What is going on? Philosophers like Maurice Merleau-Ponty, who explored this problem in the 1950s, interpreted this from the perspective of phenomenology. We see things in almost infinite diversity but never really find the reality behind the phenomena. The apparent reality constantly changes. The hand-like later stage of the disappearance of the phantom limb could be interpreted by psychiatrists as a solace for the amputee before it makes its final farewell. From neurobiologists using Hebb's perspective, the phantom limb shrinks as the nonexistent and no longer stimulated arm reduces the opportunity for reinforcing synapses that were active in the brain while the arm was in constant use. As these synaptic associations decay, the arm appears to shorten. Most of the synaptic associations are involved with the hand and not the arm itself, so those arm associations shrink first. The illusion of a caressing hand on the cheek arises, in Hebb's theory, from the random fibers of the area of the brain associated with controlling the hand being adjacent to the area of the brain associated with controlling the face. These new connections become reinforced as the arm shortens and brings the phantom hand closer to the face.

Empirical Findings of Brain Functions

From studies of stroke and accident victims, it is possible to detect where in the brain vision is associated (there are actually several parts, each of which processes a different aspect of vision, e.g., color, motion, size relationships, and perspective). Similarly, hearing and speech are located in different areas of the brain. Wilder Penfield once described a stroke victim who was an immigrant from Russia. She came to Canada as a 6-year-old child and spoke English from then on after attending school and assimilating into her new culture. After the stroke, she found her ability to speak English was lost but she could communicate in Russian. This would tell the neurobiologist that the Russian language was stored in a different area of the brain than the one damaged by the stroke. Sometimes, when brain surgery is done, a patient may be stimulated by the touch of a probe and this will evoke realistic memories of events that took place decades earlier. Neurobiologists do a lot of their studies on vertebrate brains like goldfish or mice, and they can figure out from individual neurons that are stimulated and from areas of the brain that are surgically severed or removed what motor or behavioral functions are associated with those neurons.

From physiological and biochemical studies, scientists have identified a class of compounds associated with synaptic transmission. They are appropriately called neurotransmitters and release their chemicals when stimulated by a nerve pulse. There are also compounds that specifically stimulate pleasurable responses in appropriate neurons. These are called endorphins. Opiates and other drugs popular with those who seek a chemical means of experiencing pleasure or blocking pain will often be used illegally. Unfortunately, many of these endorphin-mimicking compounds are addictive, and they can cause considerable changes in behavior and even lead to death from overdoses. Note that our understanding of how the brain works also makes us aware of the direct connection between neuronal function and human behavior. The mind is not something outside the material world. It does not coexist with the brain. If you damage the brain, you damage the mind. When neurons die, or if synapses become unwired, skills are lost. When drug abuse occurs, damage to the mind occurs. It is not guilt or some inserted member of the devil's underworld that is tweaking or corrupting that person's conscience. It is a repeatable physiological event that leads to damage and that can be studied under controlled laboratory conditions.

Neurobiology is still a young science and has a lot to learn—especially the ways that genes produce and regulate the brain. Enough is known, however, to make me wonder why this aspect of our human condition is not better known to young people. I suspect it is because most educators, religious leaders, politicians, and members of the media are as ignorant of science as the young people about whose mental health they are concerned. I once did a series of experiments in the late 1960s to test LSD on fruit flies to see if this compound (which superficially resembled a chemical I was using as a mutagen) had any genetic effects. My students and I injected male flies with an immense dose (several hundred times a human trip dose in concentration) of LSD and then used standard genetic tests for gene mutations, chromosome breakage, and chromosome loss among their descendants. We found none. Not once did I feel tempted to try LSD on myself, even if LSD had no harmful genetic effects. I reasoned that my mother was a paranoid schizophrenic and if I was heterozygous for her genes (assuming it is a genetic condition), I would be tempting fate because my threshold to such drugs might be much lower and my response more severe. When you think of your mind as a product of your neurons you have a respect for the damage products can do to the mind when they interfere with or inappropriately stimulate your neurons. How do you know what new wiring will persist? How do you know what such products might do to the capacity of neurons to generate fibers and find their connections? When you are aware of your self as existing at both the level of a social conversation and the level of cells and molecules, you take a more guarded view of tinkering without some sort of hesitation based on knowledge.

A Theory of Mind Worth Following

My colleague, Paul Adams at Stony Brook University, has been developing a theory of mind that draws analogies from Darwinian evolution and molecular genetics. He calls his model synaptic Darwinism. One theory of how life may have evolved in its earliest stages assumes that RNA evolution preceded DNA evolution. The same code applies to both of these nucleic acids, but RNA has sequences that act as enzymes. For this reason, RNA is believed to be older than DNA. DNA is more efficient because it is less subject to damage. If a gene is damaged by the excess mutations it accumulates, it cannot function. This led not only to DNA life replacing most of RNA life (RNA life today only exists among some viruses), but to longer strings of genes that had the double advantage of carrying out more functions but also allowing for more mutations, some of which were adaptive. The next great advance was the development of sexuality (in a geneticist's thinking, sexuality is the capacity of genes to combine by bringing them together into one organism from two different parents). Accompanying these many events were molecular tools for repairing damaged genes. This led to mutations, most of no benefit to survival; but occasionally a mutation added to or increased the efficiency of functions necessary to the survival of the virus (or eventually the cell).

In Adams's model, a similar process has to take place in the nervous system. The synapse is the equivalent of the gene. The sprouting of new fibers is analogous to mutations. The reinforcement by Hebbian firing together is like natural selection. There is a preservation of some neural networks and a loss of many others. The genome of a human requires about 25,000 genes. The 100-billion neurons produce hundreds of trillions of connections giving us an illusion of infinite variety that distinguishes not only one person's mind from another's, but also the year-to-year changes in our own minds. Most of this occurs in a particular part of the brain that is well-developed in humans and absent or much more modest in the brain anatomy of other animals. It is called the neocortex. This is, in Adams's model, where the uniquely human mind resides or emerges.

In science, not all theories meet the challenge of experimentation and new observations. Neurobiology has a long way to go before it can describe memory, logic, creativity, or, of unusual interest to us, our sense of self at a molecular level. To scientists, it will be a thrill if this happens. To those wedded into first- and second-millennium habits of thinking, it would be a horror. They would be frightened by it because synaptic Darwinism is such a reductionist approach to the mind. Yet, the reductionist approach to heredity has been enormously successful in working out the molecular basis of diseases such as sickle cell anemia or cystic fibrosis.

Does this reductionist interpretation of a disease offend the sensibilities of even the most religious family whose children are at risk for sickle cell anemia? It provides opportunity for prevention by prenatal diagnosis and elective abortion and it allows opportunities for a limited treatment for those for whom elective abortion is not an option, and it provides hope that a more permanent gene replacement therapy (by introducing normal genes into a child's cells taken from the child's bone marrow) can someday be added to molecular medicine.

No matter what the birth defect, once it is analyzed to the molecular level, it can lead to new treatments and opportunities to diagnose it. Most physicians welcome that experimental analysis because it adds to medical knowledge. I expect much the same will happen if Adams' model of the neocortex eventually merges with the genomic analysis of our 25,000 genes, some 5000 or 6000 of which may be associated with the nervous system. In this third millennium, we can look forward to a molecular theory of mind. It will not reduce us to automatons. There will be no sonnets found in Shakespeare's DNA. The self can never be reconstructed from the genome. We know that from the study of identical twins who can act as two different people with different minds and, not infrequently, having different careers and personalities. What makes each individual's mind unique is the capacity of the neocortex to make unique networks of Hebbian synapses in response to the input of the world that flows into each of us in uniquely different ways. With trillions of possible connections at any one time and with these connections constantly undergoing change, there is no remote possibility of two people on earth developing the same sense of self. Our minds are even more unique than our genomes.

Recommended Reading

Francis Crick's *The astonishing hypothesis* is a plea for science to use the neurobiology approach and work it to a molecular level (1994. Scribner, New York). He shows how our vision is constructed by the activities of several different areas of the brain.

PART 3

How Should We Perceive Humanity
in the Third Millennium?

THE SEVEN CHAPTERS THAT FOLLOW ALLOW US to make use of what we have learned about the biology of being human and relate it to the more traditional liberal arts approach to our identity as human beings. In Part 2, I presented a case for the unmistakable biology that governs our lives and expresses itself in birth defects, our life expectancy, our means of staving off early and unnecessary death, preventing epidemics, thwarting a variety of risks that can give us cancers, shorten our breaths, debilitate our kidneys, or render us unconscious from a heart attack or stroke. These are not trivial concerns. At the same time, I have pointed out that the biological contribution to our understanding of the human condition gives us the knowledge we need to engage in civilization without wrecking our environments or imperiling opportunities to use our talents. It is science that is our best foe of racism, sexism, and class prejudice. It exposes the fallacies of those who preserve, flaunt, and promote their privileges that often rest on bad values or bad science.

The scientific outlook I describe for the third millennium also gives us an opportunity to celebrate life, especially our own humanity. Our DNA contains a history that would fill many encyclopedias of our past ancestry and our many potentials, most of them not exercised because we are ignorant of what we are and what we can become through a knowledge of our biology. It is a field still in its infancy or gestation. Let us call it the molecular biology of the human condition. This is far from being scientism; rather, it is a liberation from the low expectations that most of humanity has assigned to others or even itself. When we are weighted down with original sin or consider ourselves innately "brutish," we begin life with such low expectations. We rely on a source other than ourselves, whether it is called societal restraint, grace, absolution, or being born again. Those ideas appeal to people who are unaware of how much good they can do for themselves or humanity by tapping into the potentials that they have. This is as true for the religious as the nonreligious. Many a preacher has offered the advice, "God helps those who help themselves."

I show that such potentials cannot be realized without recognition of what the liberal arts have provided. We are moral beings as well as biological beings. To be fully human, we have to act with those liberal arts traditions that give us dignity, a community, and a recognition or pursuit of the "good, the true, and the beautiful." We do this mostly through the Golden Rule when we do it most effectively. We betray that Golden Rule when we act out of banal self-interest or for a higher cause that uses bad means (killing, enslaving, imprisoning, exiling, intimidating, lying to, torturing, or exploiting others) to justify its ends.

CHAPTER 12

The Blank Slate, the Human Nature, and the Biological Determinism Fallacies

Do NOT JUMP TO CONCLUSIONS about this chapter's intent. I claim that there are three, almost ideological, positions about human behavior that in their more extreme forms are false. One is the idea that everything in human behavior is learned. The second is that there is a defined human nature on which science agrees. The third is that considerable human behavior (especially dealing with our culturally familiar sex, personality, and intelligence) is innate. The first is sometimes called the tabula rasa or blank slate position, the second is called the human nature argument, and the third is called biological determinism. Each has its own set of assumptions and uses different evidence to support its merits. There is no name for what I (and many others who have reflected on this problem) describe as the factors associated with the human condition.

The Blank Slate Fallacy

The blank slate is easy to grasp. A mind is likened to a computer freshly purchased. It has a mechanism analogous to a brain that sorts things into files or activities associated with the computer's storage, memory, or set aside functions. The external world or user sends in information that is unique to the computer. It may be correspondence, drafts of articles, reports, or books; it may include important photographs, music, or similar interests of the user that constantly accumulate. We would say that what the user has introduced is analogous to what we call a mind, full of knowledge, memory, discarded material, and useful programs that can carry out a variety of activities. These programs, if not introduced by the manufacturer before the user begins unpacking the computer, are produced by software installed in the computer.

In the blank slate, the brain receives sense data and shunts it to appropriate places in the brain, and by a process analogous to epigenetic development in an embryo, a sense of self emerges and an infant begins to shape and distinguish itself from a world that extends beyond the crib. For blank slate advocates, personality, sexual orientation, gender roles, intelligence, creativity, drive, and other aspects of the self are due to chance environmental stimuli as well as formal efforts by the parents to educate the child. This environment is also claimed to be complex and not fully repeatable or experienced by any two people, so even identical twins become two persons with potentially different interests and personalities even if raised in the same household.

Evidence Used by Blank Slate Advocates

Before the nineteenth century, most people in the world were either illiterate or educated to a proficiency in simple reading, arithmetic, and writing. There were no public secondary schools. There was a huge gap between the education available to the wealthy or middle class and the education for peasants, laborers, and the poor in general. Because there were so few of the elite, education in the Middle Ages was largely restricted to the clergy and royal families. In the Renaissance, wealthier merchants began hiring tutors for their children. At the time of the formation of the United States of America, education through the sixth grade was typical (there was usually a community effort to establish a one-room school house) for all except a small portion of Americans who attended liberal arts colleges or specialty schools—conservatories (for the arts), normal schools (that taught teachers), or mechanical institutes (that taught engineering). Most lawyers and doctors learned their trade through apprenticeship with practicing professionals. Most liberal arts schools were also seminaries for the religious group affiliated with their founding. Few liberal arts colleges were secular. It was widely believed that most people were incapable of benefiting from a college education.

Those views died in the last third of the nineteenth century as secondary education began to develop and secular colleges were established through acts of Congress during the Lincoln administration. Colleges for agricultural and engineering students established in the individual states also taught liberal arts students. Tuition was free or affordable for a larger segment of American students. Free secondary school education (the high school) also mushroomed in the last decade of the nineteenth century despite predictions that for most students, such required education was a waste of time.

This brief overview of how America educated its students after dissolving its colonial status with Great Britain suggests that the overwhelming majority of children born are capable of at least a secondary school education. Today, we extend that belief to college education. Note that at one time, far less than 10% of humanity was believed intellectually capable of a college education. We know that is false.

Blank slate advocates also claim that some social environments shape the beliefs of its citizens through indoctrination and cultural traditions. Spartans were raised as warriors. Athenians were more diverse in their interests. Yet both Spartans and Athenians were of close genetic identity. During the Middle Ages, it was almost universally believed that this earthly life was only of significance in determining how we were judged by God. Many Hindus have adopted a fatalistic attitude toward life and accepted their caste status because of a strong belief in the temporary nature of what we call reality and which they consider to be an illusion. Reincarnation to a higher or lower state in the next generation was a way of coming to terms with one's unhappy circumstances. There are nations where education is equated with memorizing the Koran and very little secular education is provided. Such children have a different view of their lives than do those educated in secular democracies.

Explaining Extremes of Behavior

If all people at birth have the potential to be anything their parents hope for, what causes some people to be slow or mentally retarded or inept at learning? Our views on those who do poorly in school or on achievement or intelligence tests have changed over the years. In past popular cultures, there were village idiots recognized and tolerated as part of the community. In an era when most of humanity was illiterate, it was more difficult to identify who was dull, but the very retarded made their presence known. Classifying people into psychological levels of ability was a nineteenth-century invention. Before that classification, school children who did not do well were thought to be lazy and were frequently beaten and made examples (wearing the dunce's cap) of in the classroom. After IQ (intelligence quotient) tests were introduced, students were labeled by their scores. The bell curve distribution of these scores suggested a genetic model of numerous genes acting cumulatively. At one end were those with the "smart" gene preponderance producing geniuses and at the other end were a paucity of genes for learning. This coexisted with an alternative Mendelian model that assumed there were normal people and others who carried a recessive (or dominant) gene leading to mental retardation. A third model of innate intelligence predated the idea of hereditary units and was more widely in vogue in the last half of the nineteenth century. It assumed that the protoplasm itself was defective and contaminating in those who were social failures and that retarded individuals produced retarded offspring and normal people produced normal offspring. They all shared a belief that these retarded individuals were a menace to society and should be isolated from normal people by institutionalizing them in asylums or (after 1909) sterilizing them.

By the 1930s, it was evident that mentally retarded children involved many different causes. Some were associated with the birthing process (especially near asphyxiation). Some were inherited. Some were brain damaged by injury (especially in forceps deliveries). By the 1980s, there was consensus that there were dozens of ways children could become mentally retarded. Some have an extra chromosome (Down syndrome), some have a defective gene on the X chromosome (Fragile X syndrome), some are Mendelian recessive (phenylketonuria), and some are Mendelian dominant (Apert syndrome). There is still no direct evidence for a multigene model of mental retardation, at least for IQ scores below 50.

There is less hard evidence for attributing genetic factors for very high intelligence (146 and up) in the genius category. Studies of such families do not show a discernible pattern of inheritance. The fact that eminent people produced gifted or above-average but not genius-level offspring suggested to Francis Galton that there was a regression to the mean. This is possible in multigene models of intelligence, but it would not be seen in monogenic Mendelian or X-linked inheritance. If genius had no genetic component, what then causes genius? Some geniuses are born and raised in modest households where neither parent has the education or unusual talents to serve as a model for the developing child and neither parent can think of an environmental factor that made the child so scholarly. Blank slate advocates are likely to blame bad social environments on poor achievement in students and they are probably right for most of those children. But why are there a few who do not respond that way to meager environments and instead, to everyone's surprise, excel? The reverse is also true, and many a wealthy parent has spent money on tutors to try to bail out a child who does poorly in school.

What Factors Do Show an Innate Basis?

It is evident that there are chromosomal disorders that lead to behavioral changes. Children born with XYY conditions are more likely to be overrepresented in institutionalized settings, either mental asylums or prisons. It is not that they are, on average, duller than normal males. Individuals with XXY chromosomes have Klinefelter syndrome, which makes them duller, but such individuals are not overrepresented in prisons. Down syndrome (trisomy 21) adults are usually mentally retarded and most have difficulty managing a checkbook or reading a newspaper. They frequently earn a living in supervised jobs. Genetic defects such as the Fragile X syndrome have both physical and mental abnormalities. They tend to be mentally retarded. We can argue that there are innate pathological conditions that can have effects on learning and personality. Some of the changes in behavior are striking, like the rocking back and forth on their knees and hands by children with phenylketonuria or the self-mutilation of biting fingers, lips, and tongues of children with Lesch-Nyhan syndrome, a biochemical disorder of purine metabolism producing a severe gout. The more ordinary adult-onset gout has long been associated with behavioral changes and episodes of madness. There are porphyrias that lead to madness, and George III suffered from such a genetic disorder and bouts of insanity. What these pathologies show is that the brain is not responsive to words alone. Hormones and metabolic chemicals can influence their function.

Blank slate advocates might concede such pathologies do exist and do cause mental disturbance, but they are skeptical that, in the normal functioning human brain, there are genetic or prenatal hormonal differences leading to more or less aggressive behavior, kinship bias, gender roles, sexual orientation, or a host of personality and talent differences. In this respect, neither side can be said to be right. The genetic evidence is missing. It is assumed or inferred by analogy to animal studies, by analogy to bell-shaped curve distributions, by use of twin studies (which are plagued with difficulties in controlling for extraneous factors), and by anecdotal instances that support such claims (like the choice of brand of beers or cigarettes by identical twins raised apart). The only reason pedigree studies are absent from these studies is that they were badly abused in the first third of the twentieth century when the Eugenics Record Office at Cold Spring Harbor, New York, compiled them for traits such as carpentry, seafaring, acquiring wealth, wanderlust, and other traits.

For the past 20 years, blank slate critics have used a different approach, stressing an inferred innate basis to traits that allegedly had adaptive functions in human evolution as we shifted from ape-like ancestors. These include a kin-based tribal association with an accompanying fear of outsiders and a fear of certain animals like snakes or spiders that may have arisen because many were poisonous. It also includes territoriality, because the clan or community protected its staked-out area which was its major basis for making a living by gathering and hunting in familiar grounds. It also includes a bias to one's own children or the children of closer relatives as a way to perpetuate one's own genes, an alleged basic unconscious drive in humans associated with their reproduction. The cruel treatment of children (e.g., Cinderella and Snow White) in fairy tales by stepmothers is a reflection of this alleged bias against the nonkin genes. There are even some who advocate an innate need to seek the divine as a coping mechanism for life. The study of animal behavior is not clouded with the confusion associated with human-learned behavior. The learned behavior is far less in these animal studies, and courtship rituals or dominance hierarchies are likely to be genetic in birds, deer, sea lions, and other animals studied. In fruit flies, these rituals are performed without the flies ever having seen any adults prior to their introduction to each other. You can actually map such courtship genes in fruit flies.

Resolution of what is innate in human social behavior will not occur until those genes involved in them are identified and mapped and their functions worked out. Knowledge is earned over generations or even over millennia, but humans do not usually live more than three generations, and although they are active in their careers and rearing families, they are likely to be impatient with the response, "we don't know," and would prefer the take-charge response that a trait is innate or that a trait is acquired through environmental circumstances.

The Human Nature Fallacy

The biological connection between the neurons of our brains and our capacities for numerous physical and mental skills connected to behavior is rarely denied by those who favor a blank slate. They object to more restricted social behaviors being highly directed by our neurons from birth, rather than by imprinting after birth, where it takes place in infancy or over a longer period of mental development in childhood and adolescence. One such area of dispute involves what is called human nature.

Just as the human condition changes over time in a demonstrable way, because we have a detailed historical record of how people lived and died in the past and what their expectations were, there is some evidence that views of human nature vary with past assessments of what it meant to be human. Human nature for those in the biblical tradition is perceived as seriously flawed from the beginning, with Adam and Eve showing disobedience as their first effort (after eating the apple) to shift from pet-like naïve organisms in a Garden of Eden to flawed humans who have a desire to think and reason like God. It is an ambivalent assessment because few people would have wanted to retain that status of a contented house pet. We value our ability to overcome setbacks, to experience novelty, and to trust our judgments in solving problems. There would have been no bible, no history, and a restricted range of emotions and expectations without the gift of reason provided by the eating of the fruit of the tree of knowledge.

Christian theology added a component not explicitly stated in the book of Genesis. This is original sin, a state of being that could only be circumvented by the grace of God. The easiest way to do this was through baptism. The tendency to stray from virtue after baptism suggests that the process of counteracting sin is temporary and requires renewal through the priests of the church. Catholic doctrine handled the problem of human behavioral imperfection by absolution from sins after their confession. Protestants solved the problem by accepting humans as sinners who needed prayer as a way to gain God's Grace. Piety, prayer, and a fervent desire to have those sins taken away by surrendering to God's will (especially accepting Jesus as one's savior) is a Protestant tradition to address backsliding and guilt. These religious perceptions of human nature have seen humanity as placed on earth to live out a tested life that will be weighed for future judgment with damnation (for the failures) and heavenly rewards (for the pious). Meditation, inner spiritual struggle, and atonement are other responses from other religions to address what is universally recognized in all cultures. Some people harm others by misbehaving. Some people sicken themselves with feelings of guilt for having hurt others. Not all bad acts deserve expulsion from society or being killed by the legal process that governs that society. We seek redemption for some who have erred, but in others, we feel the wrong is too grievous to be forgiven and punishment is demanded.

The Shift to a Secular Human Nature

As science emerged in the sixteenth century and began to intrude into a study of the human body, it became apparent that we were like animals in our body composition. Philosophers began to think of the mind as something independent of the soul. Very clearly, the mind went through a developmental cycle as did the body. Children did not have an innate sense of virtue. They had to learn through praise and punishment from parents, teachers, and peers that some behaviors are inappropriate in public or private. There were limits on what they could have access to. They learned about property. They learned about theft. They learned about lying. They learned about hurting others. They learned to socialize in a community in an acceptable way. Deviations from these virtues were punished by ostracism, physical beatings, or a tongue lashing to penetrate to the emotional feelings of the errant child. Children learned they could lose their privileges as well as their self-esteem.

If the mind was pliable, what did it possess? Many believed that there was a shared human nature. Some saw this as a tendency to evil that society kept in check. Some saw this as being born virtuous and then corrupted by society. Some saw this tendency as merely a potential to learn and how we turned out was not innate but a reflection of our luck in having caring parents or a caring community. It was not until Darwin studied the expression of emotions in animals that some scientists shifted their thinking away from a blank slate that is infinitely malleable to a mind restricted by its evolutionary past. In the late nineteenth century, one such belief was atavism. Humans had an alleged tendency to revert to a primitive animalistic behavior if their heredity was unfortunate enough to have such innate tendencies. We see the Robert Louis Stevenson story of Dr. Jekyll and Mr. Hyde as aspects of this atavistic murderous animal within the respectable Dr. Jekyll and expressed as the notorious criminal and killer Mr. Hyde.

In the early twentieth century, Freud presented us with a triune mind of id, ego, and superego. Their functions he assigned to a nearly forgotten or repressed past behavior of sons killing their fathers and mating with their mothers. This Oedipal interpretation of a past life, so horrible that it is cloaked in myths, is similar to the Jekyll and Hyde perception of atavisms. In both cases, no longer tolerated behaviors of the past are the source of present-day conflicts between good and evil. By the end of the twentieth century, these religious and social theories of human nature were rejected by some academics in favor of what is called evolutionary psychology.

The human nature constructed by evolutionary psychology is driven by sometimes contradictory past selection. It includes sexual selection for male behavior (typically aggressive, territorial, possessive, rational, and domineering) and female behavior (typically pacifying, social, intuitive, emotional, and supportive, but not as rational). It includes evolutionary models for kin favoritism, altruism through near-kin benefits, rejection of offspring whose paternity is suspect, and innate game theory weightings of when cheating is wise and when it is foolish. Other innate tendencies are advocated by some evolutionary psychologists for pervasive cultural beliefs such as religion. Culture acts as a brake to hereditary natural tendencies that would lead to harm, civil war, rape, pillaging, and deception on a massive scale to those who are not in one's immediate family. In this model of human nature, society is what keeps our innate tendencies muted by the greater rewards (or punishments) that unrelated society brings into being to restrain human nature.

There Are Difficulties with Evolutionary Psychology

If I did not have other alternatives, I would probably prefer the human nature of evolutionary psychologists to the religious models of original sin and its equivalents or to atavistic views of a bestial humanity repressed by modern culture or superior genes that replaced the atavistic ones. At best, I would consider evolutionary psychology a provisional theory or hypothesis. There is foremost the lack of genetic evidence for such innate traits in humans. One major failing of the eugenics movement was that its alleged and largely inferred hereditary traits leading to unfit people were spurious. Even the pedigrees accumulated by the Eugenics Record Office in the first third of the twentieth century are seriously flawed, contradicting the claims of a simple single-gene basis for social traits. Most fit a model of like-for-like inheritance that is non-Mendelian. Evolutionary psychology offers neither pedigrees nor the identification of specific genes with the numerous inferred social attributes assigned to human nature as adaptive. It might well turn out that some or most of these traits do have a genetic underpinning, but prudence would suggest that building social policy or interpreting other people's behavior on the basis of alleged innate factors is potentially dangerous, as the eugenics movement failures of the twentieth century well illustrated.

The issue of proof is independent of the issue of whether these innate traits are truly expressed. If they are, they are certainly variable in response in different cultures, different people, and different generations that it makes an innate interpretation more questionable as the basis for the failings of individuals and societies. A good deal of the evidence for evolutionary psychology is indirect and uses comparisons with animal behavior, mostly primate or mammalian. What works for gorillas may not work for chimpanzees, bonobos, gibbons, or monkeys. What works for antelopes may not apply to dogs, beavers, or a pride of lions. These animal behaviors may not, in turn, apply to us. If a well-developed capacity for reason was the most important behavior that distinguishes humans from all other animals, then we could equally invoke an evolutionary psychology interpretation that it is innate for humans to use reason whether it generates rationalizations, confabulation, outright lying, or virtuous behavior.

Let us imagine the consequences of a human nature that is innate and a human nature that is more loosely constructed primarily from cultural influences and traditions. The innate model might postulate sex differences specified earlier. As a child growing up in the 1930s, it would have appeared rational to me that women had an innate interest in child-rearing and that they avoided heavily rational fields like law, medicine, engineering, basic sciences, or business. I would have gone along with the idea that men are more aggressive and tend to like dominating other people. I would have agreed that women were innately more intuitive, in tune with their feelings, looked for social consensus, and pacified the unruly. I would have assigned that to hormones or heredity (in those days, the connections between the two were not known). If this were universally believed, there would have been no women's rights movement in the 1970s and 1980s. Those arguing for some semblance of equality in the workplace would have been told that it is a waste of time because women are not fit for such activities and would fail at it if given the opportunity to try.

It turned out that women did very well in medical school and law school and that quite a few have entered sciences. Women have entered virtually all professions that were once clubs for men. In sports, there is still a difference between males and females as professional athletes, but this may, in part, be a consequence of size and muscle development. When males are engaged in prizefighting, we do not expect a lightweight or bantamweight boxer to defeat a heavyweight champion. We match them by weight. The extra weight and muscle mass can add a lot of advantages in tennis, golf, and other sports. It may not account for all the differences between the sexes. There may be hormonal effects on muscle that testosterone has in males that makes muscle performance more effective than when it is awash in estrogens or progesterone. This could be tested. If so, then genetic differences may be less significant than hormonal differences.

But setting aside the issue of a sport's ultimate performance, the weight of the evidence is that the expectations I had in the 1930s and 1940s were shown to be false by the end of the twentieth century. When it comes to success in academic fields, it seems to be motivation, not hormones, that determines the success of those who choose that field. Curiously, today, it is males who are cited as failing more often than females in K–12 and women who are running off with the Phi Beta Kappa keys and other honors at graduation. Very few males are preaching the virtues of estrogen or an innate evolutionary need to provide a superior home life for their future children as the basis of women's academic success.

If we consider other innate traits of the first crop of evolutionary models of what makes human nature, we would include such things as aggression. At one time, modern Swedes were very aggressive (from the age of Gustavus Vasa to the death of Charles XII). Those at the receiving end of such pillaging invoked the memories of marauding Vikings and their reputation for ferocity and cruelty in the cities and villages they attacked. Their Icelandic Sagas in the tenth century provided very masculine, bloody, domineering, and hot-tempered males for their youth to emulate. But after Charles XII dominated the Baltic States and Poland and then descended into Russia (but overextended himself and went down to defeat in Poltava), he brought the remnants of his army back to Scandinavia, regrouped, and tried what he hoped would be an easier target by starting a war with Norway. A bullet through his brain ended his military adventures, and the Swedes since the early 1700s have fought in no more wars. The shift is not an infusion of cowardly or pacifist genes, but a cultural change that made Swedes tired of fighting in wars and finding it more effective to rely on manufacturing and cultivating an educated, scientific elite as models for its youth. What was once a militant society gave us the Nobel Prize for Peace (awarded, appropriately, by Norway).

If traits are inherited, we expect some sort of consistency in their expression. If the range is so broad and the environmental influence on the tendency is so powerful in shifting it about as cultural events bring about social change, then it is difficult to define the genetic trait and to distinguish it from an environmental trait that ignores any special leaning for its alleged innate potentials. Individuals may sharply differ in their personalities, career goals, choice of friends, patriotism, or capacity for empathy, but it would be difficult to imagine entire peoples sharing such traits as innate factors. The history of immigrants who came from other shores to settle in America illustrates, many times, how different are the expectations of their contemporaries when they arrive and their descendants many generations later. That was true for the immigrants who had settled into American society from the 1890s to the 1920s. They were seen as the failures of Europe who would bring down American standards in the schools and who were either condemned for living in ghettos and not assimilating or condemned for refusing to live in ghettoes and wanting to assimilate into American society. The history of exiled prisoners and paupers from Great Britain sent to Australia, with an expectation to never come back, was very similar. Those who condemned them and packed them off on ships saw them as bound to fail or create problems for the British elite sent to govern that colony.

The shift from immigrant unskilled laborers to mom and pop store proprietors to physicians and lawyers took three or four generations for those families who came to North America. Australia today has little of the outlaw image of its white ancestors.

We inherit a brain with many capacities to learn and learning is what makes us uniquely human. Learning is cumulative and it shifts us constantly away from our self-image as beasts. It often counteracts our tendency to see ourselves as burdened by human nature with guilt, sin, and a body that needs periodic scourging, for a mind whose sights should be focused on an afterworld based on faith.

The Biological Determinism Fallacy

For some time, biologists have known that mammals other than humans carry out their life cycles on automatic pilot. They have no languages written or oral. As far as we know, they do not reason or know cause and effect or go to school to learn or have communities where a huge mass of knowledge from the past is transmitted afresh each generation to young pups and cubs. Instead, they have programs that are built-in that, with a modest amount of parental guidance, get them to a point where they can survive on their own. If biologists look at animals that are not mammals, the amount of parental training is much reduced, and some invertebrates are ready to enter the adult world as soon as they hatch. The first question that comes to mind is how a brain gets programmed from birth to behave effectively for a variety of skills necessary for survival. The second question is what remnants, if any, of these "automatic pilot" skills have been passed on to us as a species, or were all of them replaced, one by one, as we made the transition from ape-like to human-like species of the genus *Homo*?

If you roll a ball bearing in front of a frog, its tongue will dart out and snatch it. It is programmed to do this whether the object is a bug, a fly, or a dirt ball. It survives because, most of the time, objects that are passing by are morsels of food. No one doubts that it is adaptive and that it is programmed rather than taught. Humans would not respond that way and we would properly assume that a different mechanism, involving thought and experience, enables us to distinguish what is food and what is dirt. Other mammals, we might surmise, have something in between. They may have built-in skills for recognizing what is living from what is flotsam if they are pulling fish out of a river. We do not have to think about what is food and what is grit when we eat; as we noted, our tongue locates the offending pebble, bone splinter, or shard of shell and navigates it to our attention and we spit it out. This is an example of being on automatic pilot for our eating habits. We may also react to sudden noises or movements, and these startle reactions may not be learned, are expressed early in babies, and happen faster than we normally reflect and then react when we deal with our conscious world.

But this is where the controversy now begins. If you discuss human behavior and classify it into sexual behavior, economic behavior, political behavior, social interaction behavior, and similar levels of discourse, there will be some biologists or social science scholars who will argue that it is all learned. Nothing is happening on automatic pilot except for what we have already learned and turned into habit or bias. Other biologists and social science scholars will argue that some of that behavior is biologically determined. Among the claims for what is biologically programmed are the following:

- Our sexual orientation—heterosexual, homosexual, asexual, or somewhere along a spectrum of attraction.
- Our gender role perception—are certain behaviors typically male (e.g., stoicism) or typically female (e.g., weeping)?
- Our personalities—friendly vs. aloof, greedy vs. sharing, self-centered vs. gregarious, timidity vs. leadership, whiny vs. composed, obnoxious vs. gracious.
- Our relation to kin—the "blood is thicker than water" perception that leads to nepotism when abused and gives relatives a special place in our feelings of caring for them.
- Our relation to nonkin—xenophobia and fear vs. welcoming and tolerance.
- Our perception of the supernatural—gullibility and a need for worship vs. skepticism or self-reliance.
- Our moral perception—retaliation and might makes right vs. empathy and practicing the Golden Rule.
- Our perception of personal space—territoriality and possessiveness vs. communal sharing.

The honest answer I give is that we do not know how much of these human interactions involve innate responses and to what degree they are programmed. I purposely paired the responses for each type of interaction because we recognize that individuals as well as cultures differ in their responses. Even the most ardent biological determinists acknowledge that gene-based expressions of behaviors fall into a range rather than narrow uniform responses. If we do consider these behavioral traits as innate, they raise difficulties for a geneticist. Are they monogenic or do they involve some sort of quantitative inheritance along a range, such as human height that usually forms a normal distribution (i.e., a bell-shaped curve)? What is the evidence? Are there distribution curves of human behavior that have been compiled? Are there other lines of genetic evidence from twin studies, adoption studies, or founder effect studies that provide support for such a genetic claim? Have psychologists devised controlled experiments to assess how such behaviors should be defined or measured? Are there studies from stroke victims and other accidents which show that such programmed behavior is lost or altered? Are there genetic syndromes with accompanying fixed social behaviors? Do such genetically disordered individuals show the same area of the brain involved as those who suffer strokes?

Why It Is Important to Have Evidence for Claims of Biological Determinism

Skepticism is an essential part of science. New claims in publications elicit skeptical responses from those in the field. They may feel that the evidence is incomplete or lacking rigor. They may feel that the experiment is flawed in design. They may feel that too much has been inferred from too little. It is part of the way science works. Others jump into the fray, do other experiments, and repeat the original experiments. Gradually, a consensus emerges that the work is solid and becomes incorporated because it passes all tests, or, if the evidence is not supportive, it remains unquoted and falls into oblivion because the work cannot be repeated or repetition leads to other interpretations that fit the data better or the alternate model makes better predictions that can be tested.

But more is at stake than good science and how it is done. Claims about human behavior have an impact on social policy. They can influence how children are taught in school. They can influence legislators on what merits financing and what merits neglect. They can create a social climate of prejudice or fear or hostility to others. They can create self-doubts and insecurity in those who believe in a judgment of their own inferiority or perversity. For centuries, African Americans felt such racist slurs, as have Jews for centuries. Ethnic insults were once accepted as valid judgments about the innate behaviors of the Irish, Italians, Slavs, Chinese, Japanese, Poles, Greeks, and Hispanics in the nineteenth and twentieth centuries.

Those who accept a strong innate component to social behaviors argue that those past assessments are racist and that ethnic slurs have no evolutionary or genetic basis and that their own work focuses on what individuals inherit and does not apply uniformly to groups. That is certainly fair enough, and I acknowledge that the vast majority of those participating in these fields that suggest a biological determinism of behavioral traits are free of that kind of overt prejudice. This may not be true of those who read of their work and use it to justify their own bigotry. Scientists are not usually held accountable for the abuses of their knowledge when that work is done as an effort to gain new knowledge. They are held accountable if that work is applied and if they are involved in those applications as consultants or participants. It suggests to me that those who publish articles about alleged innate human behavioral traits have an obligation to speak out against those who abuse that knowledge by shifting it into the realm of bigotry.

It is not just the abuse of such knowledge that is of concern to some scientists. It is difficult to tease apart what is acquired and what is inherited when a trait is described as having a range. How is that range determined? Are there environments where that range becomes fully extended and other environments where it is shortened to its full genetic expression? If a scientist cannot define the range and cannot identify how the genetic component is identified, how does that scientist distinguish such a trait from one that is picked up by psychological imprinting at an early age or one that is gradually acquired by trial and error or mimicry or the direct and indirect ways that ideas are passed on in society? In classical genetics, Wilhelm Johannsen in about 1902–1910 used a quantitative trait, bean size, and used selection to establish large bean size through inbreeding of the largest bean of each generation. After some 10 generations, he obtained a pure line in which selection no longer worked. He had established a genetically determined range and any bean, large or small within that pure line, would repeat the curve for its range when tested. Johannsen's work demonstrated that ranges of gene activity (which are genetic limits on environmental influence) can be detected through careful breeding analysis. No such experiment is possible in humans and indirect studies would be necessary. But have those studies or experiments on humans been done for claims of kinship studies, territoriality, xenophobia, or gender roles in these various attempts to isolate vestiges of past biological determinism still operating in humans?

Human Intelligence Is Difficult to Assess

Most of the controversy on biological determinism has been focused on human intelligence. This would not be much of a problem if it were a squabble about genius and its relation to intelligence testing. Intelligence testing also identifies who is incapable of learning effectively. When it is applied to the poor, to races, to ethnic groups, or to working-class children, it can reveal that they score lower on such standardized tests. The controversy involves genetic interpretations (claims from 50–90% of the determining factors involve genetic components) of a measure called the IQ score. From about 1910 to the 1960s, IQ scores were widely used by schools to sort students into three categories. A small percentage were classified as gifted or geniuses, and in more affluent school districts, there were special classes for them that gave more challenging material for them to read. The IQ was distributed in a large population as a bell-shaped curve with the mean at 100. Scores below 86 were considered slow, retarded, or worse (down to idiocy and imbecility). Scores above 115 were in the gifted category or genius category (geniuses were usually identified as 146 and higher).

The IQ test was widely abused in the years it was in vogue. Some teachers who had access to the individual records would form higher or lower expectations before the students were even in their classes. Gifted students who did a lot of the volunteer clerical work would look up their own and their classmates' IQ scores (as I and my friends did in our high school). Some corporations used IQ testing as a criterion for hiring. When I was a premedical advisor at UCLA in the 1960s, the IQ score was entered from the students' high school transcripts to the university's internal transcripts and it was available to medical admissions committees. When I did a tabulation of factors associated with medical school admissions, I found that the IQ score correlated highest with acceptance to medical school (at UCLA at that time, the mean IQ of accepted students was 135). This might suggest that it was correlated with academic achievement (or potential) or that it was of special influence to medical admissions members who had faith in the potentials claimed for IQ scores. It outranked grade point average in those days.

The greatest abuse came when IQ scores were related to class, ethnicity, and race. African Americans, Hispanics, and Native Americans had, on average, a mean IQ of 85 or close to it in the 1960s and 1970s. This suggested to some educational psychologists that those minorities would benefit from a different approach to their education during the first years of their K–12 schooling. Instead of cognitive skills, they argued, they should be taught with a stress on memory skills until they were of a more advanced developmental age when they would allegedly be ready for cognitive (problem-solving) skills. For some advocates, Head Start programs were a waste of taxpayer money because the students for whom it was intended were not ready for it. The assumption made by such educational psychologists was based on Jean Piaget's analysis of how children learn. They have to be at a certain developmental age to learn specific skills. If they are taught these skills too early, they do not respond appropriately. It would be like learning to ice skate before learning to walk. It is important to recognize that good intentions, not blatant prejudice, motivated those who made these suggestions. What they did not anticipate is that some people would give up on those with lower IQ scores (or whole groups whose mean IQ score was lower than average). Underlying their motivation in making these judgments was the belief that IQ scores are fixed by heredity and nothing society could do would remedy their limited abilities to learn.

What made me skeptical about IQ scores was an incident that happened about 1970 when I was at Stony Brook University. A group of graduate students asked me if they could have some time in my class to discuss the IQ controversy. I gave them half my lecture hour. One of the speakers was an African American woman who was completing her Ph.D. She said that when she was a child, her mother was told that her daughter's IQ was 75 and that she would be placed in a class with other retarded students. Her mother replied that she knew her daughter and her daughter was not retarded and that she would take it to court if such a transfer was carried out. This very gifted graduate student said she was grateful for her mother's faith in her abilities and wondered what her life would have been like if she had been taught in classes with low expectations about her ability to learn.

There are other reasons to be skeptical about the predictive power of IQ scores. There is no doubt they correlate well with academic success. The highest IQs are found among the middle-class households where parents are educated, have a strong interest in their children's education, provide many intellectually stimulating opportunities such as educational toys, travel during vacation breaks, and participation in extracurricular activities such as music lessons and trips to libraries, bookstores, museums, and other educational facilities. Lewis Terman had a great deal of faith in the relation of IQ score to eminence in society. He identified a cohort of 1000 high school students in California with high intelligence at or near-genius level (a mean of about 140) and studied them. They were born about 1910. He followed them until he died and his students followed them until most of the cohort had died. He called his project *Genetic Studies of Genius*. Terman's kids were followed by questionnaires throughout their careers. Most came from middle-class households and entered middle-class professions, especially law, medicine, engineering, education, and business. Few entered the fine arts. Those with an interest in the humanities became college professors. They wrote a lot of books, mostly nonfiction scholarly works. They published thousands of articles in professional journals if they went into academic careers. None had a biography written about them. They were not eminent. The most successful (from a financial measure) was the inventor of the situation comedy for television.

Quite different were those twentieth-century Americans who had two or more biographies written about them and thus could be considered eminent by that standard of recognition. Victor and Muriel Goertzel studied them in the 1960s and identified some 300 persons. Their fields were similar to those chosen by Terman's high-IQ students, but there were more creative fields among them, especially in fields such as music performance, fine art painting and sculpting, and acting. The Goertzels noted several differences among them when contrasted to Terman's kids. Goertzel's cohort had more unhappy times growing up than did Terman's. The parents were divorced, widowed, or experienced business failure or one parent was psychologically stressful because of alcoholism or psychosis or just being a crank. The students were rarely teacher's pets. Many of them were bored by their K–12 experience and felt unmotivated and some were even disruptive in class. What set apart the Goertzel group was a cluster of activities that they described as intense focus, an ability to complete their projects, a passion for doing what they liked to the neglect of normal expectations of socializing with others, and unusual creativity or imagination. The mean IQ score they obtained for their cohort, from searching their school records or from interviews and correspondence, was 124.

Biological determinism becomes a fallacy when it is asserted as proven, although the evidence is indirect and subject to different interpretations. Because it is a very volatile field, extreme caution is needed to prevent abuse, misinterpretation, or exploitation by those who tuck it into their favorite biases and use it as justification of that bias. I am not arguing that biological determinism is false. The evidence to prove it false is also indirect and lacking the tough criteria of those sciences that have controlled experiments that meet the objections of their critics. But where asserted knowledge can influence public policy, it is better to be skeptical and cautious than confident or dogmatic.

Recommended Reading

This is a field with an immense popular literature. Steven Pinker's *The blank slate: The modern denial of human nature* (2002. Viking, New York) takes a dim view of that constructed view of how we behave. His book, *How the mind works*, gives an overview of the evidence for evolutionary psychology as a powerful foundation for human behavior. See also Paul Ehrlich's *Human natures: Genes, cultures, and the human prospect* (2000. Island Press, Shearwater Books, Washington D.C.) for a more diverse view of human behavior and its differences. Also see Rod Gorney's *The human agenda* (1972. Simon and Schuster, New York) for the role of "work, play, and love" as essential components of our psychic needs.

I recommend Victor and Muriel Goertzel's *Cradles of eminence* (1962. Little, Brown, Boston) for the roles that creativity, imagination, focus, and drive play in achieving eminence.

CHAPTER 13

Human Nature as Potential for Forming Communities

W HAT CONSTITUTES BEING HUMAN? All agree that the use of reason is one such component in what distinguishes us from other mammals. We use reason in a complex way that other mammals fail to match. We can use it to shape tools, to use tools to make other tools, and to imagine tools that are manufactured in ways that the material from which they are made do not suggest. A skinned animal does not suggest that it can form a hat, a jacket, or a tent. A rock does not suggest that flakes cracked off from it with another rock can be used as cutting tools to slice meat or hides. Reason does more than make tools. It permits us to have a sense of self. We become the tool user, the imaginer of how to design new tools and to use the products of our work for artificial products that enrich our lives. They can be shelters with places to sit or places to sleep; they can be clothing to warm us, or provide recognition of our status in the community; they can be barriers to keep out dangerous animals. Reason gives us an understanding of cause and effect. It allows us to figure out how the universe works.

We have other innate potentials. The capacity for language is turned on in children at an early age, and during those years, the children learn vocabulary and the specific ways words are organized in sequence to convey information. As adults, we lack that capacity and we struggle to learn a new language, often with pronounced accents. Something has changed in the way our brains work for acquiring this skill. Children also shift from the concrete to the abstract as they go through their teen years. Experiments demonstrate that a task requiring abstract thought cannot be done by most students who are younger than 18 years old. I remember seeing an educational psychologist who studied how children learn science demonstrating this. Imagine ten students given a net and they each dip it into a small pond ten times and they obtain a total of ten frogs. How many frogs were in the pond at the start of the experiment? Most first-year students are befuddled and guess. They do not know how to set up a proportion of the probability of catching a frog (1 in 10) and the proportion of found frogs to expected frogs (represented as 10 are to X). Setting this into an equation $1/10 = 10/X$ gives 100 as the answer. Piaget showed that children's perceptions of volume are not separated from size while they are preschool age. They identify the same volume of a fluid as larger if the vessel is tall and thin rather than short and shallow.

Humans Form Communities

We are not unique in forming communities. Birds often flock together. We are startled by the numerous members of herds of cattle, antelopes, elephants, giraffes, and other animals when we watch films on the migrations of these animals in Africa. How then do human communities differ from the communities of birds, fish, and animals? Human communities are dependent on learning for the success of their communities. Our capacity to learn and to use reason sets us apart. We transform our environments. Our tools can level trees. We can use fire to destroy unwanted vegetation. We can dig canals for irrigation. We can build barriers such as walls to keep out other animals or other humans. No other animal uses fire as a tool. Our communities are repositories for learned skills that do not have to be discovered anew in future generations. They are teachable. We have inherited or learned the skills of being gregarious, of living together, of craving human companionship. These tendencies are influenced by cultures. At one time, guilds were associated with kindreds. Strangers did not get to do those jobs. Today unions are not kin-dependent.

Communities also depend on trust. Humans have a capacity for trust and empathy. They can imagine situations and see themselves in a community. It is not limited to kin where bonds are built through a family in which the young are dependent on their parents and near relatives. Children have the innate skills of smiling and eliciting feelings of care and protection from adults. We feel that delight when we see a kitten or a puppy. It is much more intense with our own children when they are infants. We feel it when we see a child in a baby carriage when we stop to chat with an acquaintance.

When there is no community, children do not do well. About once a year there will be a story in the news of parents who have never sent their child to school. The child has lived in a room isolated from contact with others except for the occasional times the parents bring in food. Such children have a limited vocabulary and their learning disorders are severe. Their capacity for acquiring language skills is limited. Their emotional responses to others are poor. Whatever innate capacities we may have for being reasonable, learning, and responding to others has to be brought into reality by actual contact with others. Our innate capacities do not find expression without that exchange and opportunity to use them. It is as if they are atrophied. Infants who were neglected in institutions frequently showed symptoms of this lack of stimulus. Today, their caregivers make sure that the children are exposed to smiling faces and that the staff holds them, plays with them, and talks with them. We have potentials, but it is the appropriate environment that brings them out.

Whether we have built-in tendencies for faith in the supernatural is debatable. Most children raised without a religion or god concept learn to live with that secular world view. Human diversity assures that there will be crossover events. Some religious parents find that their children become agnostics or atheists. Some atheist parents find that their children become deeply religious. Children may have a capacity to believe what adults say because they are dependent on them and most of what they have learned from a parent has been beneficial. This is why children will accept, initially, stories of tooth fairies, Easter bunnies, Santa Claus, and other icons of childhood. If their parents treated a belief in God as equivalent to these childhood imagined beings, and dropped their beliefs when the child turned 9 or 10 by saying that this is just a childhood fiction, most children might become skeptics. We do not know if this is true because it is not something most parents would wish to put to a test. The abandoned beliefs in childhood supernatural beings are not as traumatic as abandoning a belief in God. Holidays or rites of passage are limited in number and so are the roles assigned to the mythic figures associated with them. Belief in a God is far more extensive in its effects. It helps a community face setbacks such as floods, plagues, fires, drought, and other disasters. This would have been particularly true when very little science was known about how nature works. Religious faith also helps families cope with illness and death. It helps the individual when bad things happen such as losing a job, getting injured in an accident, or seeing a marriage collapse. Restoring emotional good feelings and self-esteem is a more difficult task than fixing a leaky roof or clogged drain. Trying to reason out misery or sorrow seems like using the wrong tools for the job.

What is very difficult to reconcile in interpreting theories of human nature are the contradictions we observe in human behavior. When we think of pathological conditions associated with cell, tissue, or organ malfunction, we usually can construct pedigrees and infer the mode of inheritance. Some traits are recessive, some are dominant, and some are X-linked recessive. All are rare if they cause considerable ill health or infertility. Mild conditions like color blindness may be as high as 6% of the males in a large population like Great Britain. Other conditions involve two or more genes, and their pedigree charts are not as predictive on who will inherit a cardiac defect at birth or a neural tube defect or a cleft lip and palate. Their mode of inheritance is determined by compiling a large number of pedigrees. If the population at large has an incidence of 1 in 1000 for a cardiac defect, a healthy sibling of a person who had such a defect may have a 3% chance of passing it on. If a child had a cleft lip and palate and it was surgically repaired and if that person has a spouse and produces a child, the odds go up to about 8% of passing it on.

It is difficult to compare these multigene conditions with some inferred multigene basis for personality. How does one define and evaluate a person who is generous and a person who is a tightwad? The tightwad could be generous to family members but not to charities and strangers. People who are generous with money may not be generous with their time. Worse yet, a person may be generous in youth and stingy in middle age. This is very different from clinically defined conditions like a ventricular septal defect or pyloric stenosis. You do not flip from an anatomical lesion of the mouth to an anatomical lesion in your gut or anus. The medically defined traits are fixed and can sometimes be repaired. The psychological attributes are more difficult to pin down scientifically or descriptively. From the perspective of pedigree analysis, they are also difficult or impossible to analyze because so much of the expression of personality traits is acquired even if there are alleged tendencies in the family. This is less of a problem for psychoses such as bipolar disorders, where the clinical criteria for evaluation are very good. Even if pedigrees were not compiled, how would one classify humanity in a set of personality traits? Even a trait such as homosexuality is difficult to assess. Alfred Kinsey saw about 40% of males having had at some time in their life a homosexual experience leading to orgasm. He generated a range from 1 to 6 to classify such individuals and showed that homosexuality is a spectrum of orientation with different incidences or times of expression, but only a small percentage, about 2–3%, are homosexuals who have considered their orientation exclusively homosexual. Do heterosexuals with one homosexual experience in their youth become homosexuals for purposes of classification? Does one spot make a leopard?

Recommended Reading

Piaget introduced the idea of developmental stages in forming the mind from infancy to adulthood. See his book, *The child's construction of reality* (1955. Routledge and Kegan Paul, London). Lawrence Kohlberg used Piaget to work out the developmental stages of moral behavior. His ideas are represented in William Crain's *Theories of development*, 5th edition (2005. Prentice Hall, Upper Saddle River, New Jersey).

CHAPTER 14

Science Enriches Our Appreciation of the Arts and Humanities

I ONCE RELATED TO MY CLASS A COMMENTARY that Charles Darwin made in his short autobiography, which he wrote in the 1840s for his family in case he died prematurely from his real or imagined chronic illnesses. In it, he mentioned that as a youth he loved the humanities and memorized many passages from Shakespeare's plays and delighted in reading novels. But once he became obsessed with natural history from the time he embarked on the voyage of the *Beagle* to the time of his writing of the autobiography, he found neither time nor inclination to read in the humanities. He described the experience as a form of atrophy of his aesthetic sensibilities. One student at the end of the course said that the most frightening thing he had ever heard in my lectures was Darwin's loss of his aesthetic soul. I reassured the student and apologized that I had not added a follow-up. Darwin never revised that biography, but we know from accounts of his life for the remaining 40 years or so that he lived, he read aloud to his wife her favorite new novels and this once again ignited his aesthetic feelings, even if they did not match the passion of his youth.

One of the characteristics of driven people is that they can become monomaniacs while pursuing and completing an endeavor. If we read Dostoyevsky's account of gambling in some of his fiction, we realize that such moments can eclipse all other human interests. Dostoyevsky wrote convincingly of the experience because he was at times a compulsive gambler. Many a marriage in graduate school or in the early years of a scientific career has foundered on the work habits of the driven spouse who cannot leave the laboratory. It no doubt happens to those in law, politics, medicine, and business as well. Fortunately for Darwin, he worked at home and learned to budget his time for his wife and his family. Much more important to assess is whether a thorough knowledge of science causes a loss of interest in the arts and humanities. Most scientists would deny this and quite a few scientists, including Nobelists, have been artists, musicians, sculptors, photographers, novelists, and poets. What the most able in any field recognize is that it is difficult to spread oneself too thin. Generalists today have a tough time making major discoveries.

The Two-cultures Concern

Physicist C.P. Snow was both a novelist and a critic of contemporary culture. He created a debate in academic circles with his publication of *The Two Cultures* based on a series of lectures he gave in 1959. He argued that among his many colleagues and friends, there was a gulf between those who were in the arts and humanities and those who were in the sciences. Although scientists had a liberal arts education and some familiarity with music, fine arts, and literature, he found that very few of those who were in the arts or humanities had any knowledge of the sciences. This made them unable to participate in discussions of importance to society (he wrote the book in the early years of the Cold War and the Atomic Age). He charged universities and precollege schools with neglecting the education of those who favor a humanities or arts education. He also accused his humanities colleagues of falsely assuming that science was not relevant to an appreciation of the human condition.

From today's perspective, Snow's concern is somewhat dated. Virtually all college undergraduates in the United States are required to take one year of science (usually with a laboratory component). At the time when Snow wrote his complaint, European (and Canadian) science undergraduates had virtually no courses except those in their major field of interest and the cognate sciences they needed (for biologists that would have been chemistry, physics, and mathematics courses). Two generations have elapsed since Snow's plea was made and a lot has changed in our understanding of science and the role it has in our lives. Virtually all of molecular biology has changed profoundly how we look at birth defects, cancer, environmental mutagens, diagnostic medicine, and the modification of life by gene transfer. The attention to issues like climate change, especially global warming, loss of biodiversity, the pollution of oceans and other waters, and the expansion of weapons of mass destruction has made the need for science literacy of some kind an important concern. It is no longer a question of those in the humanities and arts giving a cold shoulder to scientists. We are all imperiled together by runaway developments of science and technology poorly regulated, rationalized by dubious values, and even encouraged, especially at a government level where the power to bring about change is essential.

How Science Influences the Arts and Humanities

The Faust legend is a good example of how science is perceived by different generations. The Faust legend began to circulate in the Renaissance. Although that legend might have begun centuries earlier among alchemists, it was often associated in Renaissance times with Paracelsus, a controversial physician and chemist (as well as alchemist). He has been described as a leader in bringing science out of the grip of magic. His unconventional life (especially the use of the vernacular instead of Latin to promote his works and his numerous attacks on academic traditions) inspired modification of the Faust legend, turning Faust into the obsessed scientist who would sell his soul for more knowledge. In Christopher Marlowe's portrayal in the 1592 *Tragedie of Dr. Faustus*, Dr. Faustus is evil and descends into a fiery hell for his 24 years of misbehavior, a version that resonated more than 200 years later when Gounod wrote his *Faust* opera. Here, the obsession is not new knowledge but the seduction and corruption of Marguerite. Here too he finds his reward in hell. Quite different from the prevailing Faust legends is the view of Johann Wolfgang von Goethe, who had no quarrel with academic learning, but who sees Faust as not only desirous of new knowledge, but having a conviction that knowledge has no limits and if he ever finds satisfaction in an activity that he wants to do as an ongoing commitment, Mephistopheles could take his soul. Goethe's Faust lives on to be 100 before he finds that commitment. It is science in the service of humanity. He becomes the engineer, the city planner, and the scientist who desires to convert swampland into harbors, farms, and healthy cities. Instead of being cast in hell for the wake of bad outcomes his life with Mephistopheles had brought about in his 50-year quest for new knowledge and experiences, he is saved by God for his good intentions and commitment in this final realization of the uses of knowledge.

Faust in Goethe's perception is an extension of the Renaissance ideal of the "universal man" who embraces all knowledge and unites the arts, humanities, and sciences. We know from Giorgio Vasari's accounts of these artists that they were enthusiastic about science because it gave them insights into perspective, new pigments to create colors, the engineering skills to cast giant statues in bronze, an anatomical knowledge to create an illusion of realism, and new tools to do art. No doubt, Goethe himself felt that way, because he began his career as a mining engineer and made contributions to botany and zoology.

Novelists like Emile Zola had a love for science and Zola would devote hours to library study and doing interviews with experts as he constructed his 20-volume series on the Rougon and Macquart families. He was stimulated by the thinking of scholars of his day on degeneracy theory and its ties to heredity. Both geniuses and psychopaths came out of his fictional families. Fyodor Dostoyevsky was also influenced by such theories of the day. In *The Brothers Karamazov,* he pits the rationalist brother Ivan and the spiritual brother Alyosha and contrasts them with their epileptic and psychotic half-brother, Smerdyakov. He also brings the clash of religion and reason into sharp contrast with one of the most famous passages in literature, Ivan's parable of the Grand Inquisitor in which Jesus returns to earth *in cognito* in hopes of making humanity use its reason as a guide to living and the Grand Inquisitor demands (and gets) an imposed authoritarian obedience to keep humanity from straying into error.

In the twentieth century, Sigmund Freud had a powerful influence on writers. D.H. Lawrence's novels reflect his interest in oedipal theories and an underlying sexual world view of humanity. The clash of science and religion, the rational and the spiritual, is well reflected in the novels of Herman Hesse. In *Narcissus and Goldmund,* the rational and ascetic Narcissus and the spiritual and emotional sculptor Goldmund see their world in conflicting ways and neither is capable of complementing the other. In Roger Martin du Gard's *Jean Barois*, there is a searching analysis of the conflict between Barois, a biologist turned journalist, and his daughter, who becomes a nun. Barois is a freethinker and learns how difficult it is to live a rational, atheistic life stripped of spirituality. He learns that the affairs of the day, including the Franco-Prussian War and the Dreyfus Affair, melt away into history while the deep needs of friendship, love, and family prevail whatever one's belief and whatever the passions of politics may be. Neither his boyhood Catholic religion nor science satisfies the aging Barois confronting his mortality.

A similar look at poetry, sculpture, and painting will show many instances where science enters into the artist's thinking and becomes transformed in aesthetic ways, sometimes celebrating science and sometimes depicting its melancholy or depravity. Goya saw nightmares coming from the "dreams of reason." Stella saw abstract beauty in his painting "Brooklyn Bridge." Brancusi reduced "Bird in Flight" into Pythagorean streamlined simplicity. Picasso delighted in hearing about the advances of science and it stimulated cubism as a way to portray reality in geometric isolates. Thomas Hart Benton's murals celebrated the sciences in numerous Depression-era murals painted in government buildings and universities. Surrealists like Remodios Varos, Rene Magritte, Salvador Dali, and Max Ernst explored science in their art. More contemporary twenty-first-century examples include musician, composer, and inventor Laurie Anderson, painter and futurist Alexis Rockman, and Matthew Ritchey, whose multimedia works and drawings are inspired by evolution and cosmology.

The Dialog of Science and the Humanities

Whatever Snow's peeve was between the circles of his scientist friends and the circles of colleagues in the humanities, there is ample evidence that science and the humanities have always been in dialog. It may not be the amount of engagement scientists desire, and it may not be as favorable as scientists might wish for. What is missing from Snow's view is the moral discourse between science and government, science and industry, and science and those who portray it to the public. When science is the obedient servant of the government, it is Goya's vision that prevails—mass murder of the innocent is not only justified but celebrated. It happened in the Third Reich. It happened at Hiroshima and Nagasaki. These events will certainly be interpreted differently by winners and losers or victims and perpetrators. We do not see the events of 9/11 as a triumph of martyrs to a higher cause. We see it as terrorism.

What unites these three historic events is their reliance on science to carry out mass murder and the impotence of science or religion to prevent it. We rely on first- and second-millennium outlooks to justify why we do horrible things, and we are like hapless people groping in the dark with both reason and religion having failed us.

Recommended Reading

C.P. Snow's contribution was *The two cultures* (1993. Cambridge University Press, London).

CHAPTER 15

Moral Values Bind a Community

IF THE HALLMARKS OF BEING HUMAN ARE BASED ON REASON and the need to be part of a community, then getting along in that community is essential. Humans also have to be moral. We do not know much about morality in the animal world because most of the behavior is on automatic pilot and not reflective. Among mammals, some sort of moral sense may prevail. One time in Kenya, my wife and I were at a national park and the van in which we were traveling came upon a cluster of elephants, about five of them, including two young ones. The matriarch of the group moved forward, lifted her trunk, blasted out a sound, waited for the van to stop, and then led the way for her group to cross the road. After they were across the road, she then raised her trunk again and honked. It felt like an act of trust. If I signal you to stop, you will respond appropriately, and we will then both go on our way. It was as if some sort of Golden Rule was in play. That might be an anthropomorphic interpretation and I am not wedded to the idea of animal morality, but it is very clear that humans do carry out acts of reciprocity as one of their moral behaviors and give names to those acts.

Humans go through a Piagetian developmental phase for their moral behavior, as psychologist Lawrence Kohlberg first pointed out. The initial acts of toddlers are selfish—they might take another child's toy without asking. As very young children learn to socialize and learn that behavior brings about responses in others, they begin to act in terms of reciprocity. Their first moral code is close to Middle Eastern behavior three or four millennia ago—tit for tat reciprocity or "eye for an eye" justice. Punch me

139

and I will punch you. Pull my hair and I will pull your hair. By puberty, children have learned the Golden Rule, "Do unto others as you would have them do unto you." This requires reason, not reaction. You have to have empathy to practice the Golden Rule. You imagine a moral universe where there is no intentional harm done to you so you do not intentionally harm others. I am not sure the negative form of the Golden Rule, popularized by Rabbi Hillel, occurs spontaneously in a child or young adult, "Do not do unto others what you would not have done unto you." It is more sophisticated because it puts limits to behavior rather than opening up the Golden Rule to some confusing aspects of reciprocity. Does the Golden Rule mean that if you are generous and like to pay the tab at dinner during a night out that you expect others to be as generous to you? Generosity may be a private virtue, but public behavior does not demand such private virtues. It demands some semblance of order, fairness, and consensus on behavior that does not harm others.

Most moral views are based on religious traditions. The Golden Rule is expressed in biblical literature. It appeared in several civilizations about the fifth century B.C.E. Before that formulation, the most frequently cited moral code in our western tradition was the Ten Commandments. It is several centuries older than the Golden Rule. It is described in the Bible as having been engraved on tablets and passed from God to Moses to give to his people. It has an authoritarian sanction. Four of these commandments deal with the relation of people to God (no other gods should be worshipped, no idols or images should be worshipped as substitutes for him, God's name should not be misused for personal purposes; and people should keep the Sabbath).

There is one commandment regulating a child's obligations to the parents (it says to be nice to them and respect them). The remaining five are cast as negatives: don't kill, don't commit adultery, don't steal, don't lie, and don't covet (envy) your neighbor's property, family, or success. For Jews and Christians, who both follow the Ten Commandments, it is a religious necessity. They are ordained by God. Despite the commandment not to make graven images, modifications have been made. Roman Catholics and most Protestants do not consider it as a graven image to have a representation of Jesus on a cross or numerous works of art depicting the stages of his life. Virtually all nations, no matter how religious they may be, will allow killing in times of war and for numerous other circumstances from self-defense to killing those who blaspheme God. For some theologians, the Ten Commandments do not apply to those who worship other gods or who are nonbelievers. You can lie or steal when dealing with them; you can also kill them.

Humans are very inventive and they can come up with end runs around almost any commandment. Adultery is avoided by having divorce or annulment to end a marriage. Adultery is avoided by having multiple wives, a practice that is accepted in the Biblical literature. Adultery is avoided by designating a woman as a concubine. People who "keep up with the Joneses" do not think of themselves as covetous. They think of themselves as hard-working Americans looking for a better life. When governments lie, they call it spin. When a company declares bankruptcy to get rid of its obligations to pay health insurance or pay pensions already contributed by its workers, or contractually promised to them, it does not think of it as stealing those funds. It describes its actions as "restructuring" and goes on bringing in profits to its stockholders.

Moral Codes Can Be Based on Reason Instead of Faith

I am struck by how many people tell me that without a belief in God, there would be no moral standards and everything would descend into the chaos of relativity. Morality may have been the exclusive right of religions to teach in ancient times, but just as their hold on interpreting the universe gave way to the development of science, morality has also been the subject of philosophic analysis. It can be based on reason.

Immanuel Kant proposed an empathy-based test of morality. He argued that if a reasonable person asked "Do I want anyone to kill me?" the reasonable person would say no. If all reasonable persons said the same thing, then killing is universally recognized as immoral and should not be done. The same line of argument would be applied to stealing, lying, or fornicating (by someone else) with one's spouse. I am not sure coveting would have met Kant's test because a reasonable person might tolerate another person's envy rather than condemn it. I also think that the religious obligations about God would not meet Kant's standard because reasonable people tolerate atheists, agnostics, and deists who would have been condemned by a Ten Commandments standard. Similarly, graven images would have little impact on Kant's reasoning sane people. Some would have accepted it as artistic expression or part of another person's faith whose practices they would tolerate.

There is another secular moral guide that is sometimes expressed by the phrase "Virtue is its own reward." This is not a concept a child can grasp. Adults who reflect on that phrase (as I did from the time I was in grade school and befuddled by that phrase prominently displayed above the blackboard) realize that it is a nice way to live in a community with others. You do not do good things in expectation of reciprocity. You do good things because they are right and you feel good about it. Reciprocity has an element of selfishness to it. It is lower down in Kohlberg's ranking of how to behave. Doing good as part of your being or world view is an expression of what it means to be fully human. You are in tune with your capacity for empathy. You may not intend it, but your acts may be a model for others. I remember looking out the window of the old biology building when I was a graduate student and studying in the library at Indiana University. A sudden shower was drenching the parking lot and there, in shirtsleeves, moving rapidly from car to car was Ralph Cleland. He was rolling up the windows that his colleagues had left down. Ralph Cleland was a member of the National Academy of Science, Chair of his department, a botanist of renown, whose evolutionary studies of the evening primrose *Oenothera* were a classic, and who was deacon of his Presbyterian Church. I admired that act of virtue, doing the right thing because Cleland was that sort of person.

Whether morality is reason-based or faith-based, it is essential for us to be moral beings. Communities can only work with some guarantee that its members do not have to worry about being killed, robbed, deceived, or lied to. The great difficulty of all moral systems, however motivated or whatever their historical origin, is the lack of consistency in applying them. Kant took great pains to insist that "no exceptions" should be made to his moral imperatives. Later, he made exceptions. Without exceptions, there would be no wars. Without exceptions, there would be no capital punishment for heinous crimes. Without exceptions, you would have limited options (with odds against survival) if you were attacked. In the film based on the story of Sergeant Alvin York, a hero of World War I, York begins as a fundamentalist youth who was a crack shot hunter and the male equivalent of an Annie Oakley in his rural community. He at first refuses to be inducted in the army because of his beliefs taught by his church that he "shall not kill." Patriotism eventually trumped those religious commandments, and in the movie, he uses deception to lure German troops into view and he kills them in large numbers. The audience cheered during that scene. What is going on? The country who celebrated his heroism a generation earlier did not see Sergeant York as evil, nor did those watching the movie. Most of the congregations in the nation would have seen him as a Christian in good standing when he returned to civilian life.

Sergeant York shows the dangers of a reason-based moral code that has done more harm to humanity than any other moral code. It is called utilitarian ethics. It was given that name in the early nineteenth century by Jeremy Bentham and endorsed by John Stuart Mill as a democratic ethic in which the greatest good is done for the greatest number. It sounds nice, but it has a potential for mischief. It works by invoking a higher cause as an escape clause from rights-based ethics, whether the Ten Commandments, the Golden Rule, or Kantian imperatives. With utilitarian ethics, you can argue that dropping the atomic bomb on Hiroshima will save more lives than it kills because (here comes the higher cause) it will end the war more quickly. With utilitarian ethics, you can say that the state can sterilize the unfit people who are sapping its resources because (again the higher cause) it will cleanse the nation of its degenerates. Those degenerates can then be paupers, criminals, psychotics, and the retarded, or, if you elect killing instead of sterilization, they can be Jews, gypsies, Slavs, and homosexuals. Horrible crimes become moral acts with a simple invocation of a higher cause. People kill in God's name (despite the commandment not to invoke God's name in vain). They kill for patriotism. They kill for ideology. They kill for the honor of their family.

Some biologists would argue that human nature makes consistent morality impossible. They would claim that kinship-loyalty leads to killing nonkin unless it is held in check by punishments. They would claim that innate aggression in males makes them natural warriors. What is unnatural, for such perceptions of human nature, is loving one's neighbor like oneself. Many religionists would also argue that people are prone to doing harm to others because of their sinful birth. Their life on earth is a way to play out the choices of evil acts or acts of goodness so that they can be judged for their fate in an afterlife.

All societies have worked out a system of rewards and punishments for public behavior. Those who harm others are usually punished by state institutions, usually courts and a legal system. In times past, it might have been a King or a tribal leader who listened to the evidence.

In biblical times, it might have been the adult males who listened to accusations, rendered a judgment, and then stoned to death a person convicted of a capital crime or expelled a person from the community if it were a lesser crime.

The search for the ideal society or the ideal moral code cannot be realized because of our diversity. Being human may include vague feelings of empathy and other virtues. But being human also may include vague feelings of envy, anger, or aggression. Whether those vague feelings arise out of the diverse experiences of growing up or out of some ancestral adaptive behavior engraved into our psyches by our genes is still much in dispute. We may not know why we are moral animals, but we know that no society can exist without a moral code.

Recommended Reading

Moral values are significant in all aspects of life. Some theologians and philosophers have made a specialty of scientific ethics. Just as religious traditions run from liberal to conservative, so do these ethical interpretations of science. On the liberal side is Lee Silver's *Challenging nature: The clash of science and spirituality at the new frontiers of life* (2006. Ecco, New York), and on the conservative side is Leon Kass's *Toward a more natural science: Biology and human affairs* (1985. Free Press, New York).

CHAPTER 16

The Human Condition and Our World Views Change Every Generation

I AM NOW THREE GENERATIONS OLD. My first generation (1931–1956) carried me from the Great Depression (technically, I was born as a Hoover baby) and World War II until the heyday of the Beat Generation. My second generation (1957–1982) carried me through the 1960s and its powerful influences on young people, making them aware of civil rights, women's rights, and patients' rights. My third generation (1983–2006) was more disappointing politically because it offered greed as a virtue, a huge chasm between the rich and poor fostered by tax cuts for the rich, and lost opportunities in a world that saw the death of Communism and the Cold War by an unexpected self-implosion. This is just one lifetime nearing its end. The science, music, art, movies, novels, journalism, theatre, eating out, transportation, and expectations are profoundly different in these three generations. What has changed is the human condition.

Consider life expectations. Growing up poor in New York City, the son of an elevator operator, in slummy neighborhoods rich with roaches and bedbugs, I saw my future in those slums. The Depression offered few hopes to the poor. It offered relief but no way out. It was not a miserable life. The museums were free and I could learn to appreciate the art and civilizations on display at the Metropolitan Museum of Art. I learned to love the natural history on display in the American Museum of Natural History with its dioramas and its display cases of the diversity of life on earth. Central Park was free, and even if I could not play with a sailboat like those the rich boys brought down to sail in the pond near East 70th Street, I could enjoy seeing them glide triumphantly in the water. Being poor did not deprive me of painting in watercolors or reading avidly. I did not know until I was in high school that I could attend college. (I got a scholarship to New York University.) I did not know shortly after I entered high school that the field I loved, genetics, required a Ph.D. or that such a degree existed. I was lucky because I was a scholar and my teachers steered me to an academic life. For most of my classmates, high school graduation was the end of the line. They had no money for college and those that were desirous faced too high an academic bar for them to leap over.

For the second of my generations, things changed dramatically. Colleges had expanded in number and size, mostly thanks to the GI Bill, which opened college to the ordinary citizen. It required military service, but virtually every young male who turned 18 between 1940 and 1945 was drafted into the army. They led the way. When I entered college in 1949, I was not a novelty; lots of GIs were still in attendance. They showed that they could handle college as effectively as the sons of the privileged. There were fewer women going to college then so I use the masculine because it describes the expectations of that generation. Women got married. Husbands were breadwinners. There was a rebellion brewing with my fellow students, who were turned off by the dull normality of suburban life that was taking place ("men in gray flannel suits"). They did not see themselves as carrying briefcases to and from commuter trains. They wanted the open road. They were disillusioned that peace had turned into a Cold War and a Korean War. Soon they would be in a Vietnam War. They were disillusioned that so little progress was made to end the discrimination that lingered on from the Civil War a century before. They sought change through civil rights movements and joined voter registration drives. We shifted our expectations from individuals who served institutional ideologies and prejudices to individuals who asked that their autonomy be respected. It extended from African Americans to women. It extended to the entire health field, and paternalism in medicine shifted abruptly as patients demanded to know more about their problems and treatment options that were available to them. Autonomy crushes humility and deference.

My children grew up in my second generation, and all of their classmates knew from an early age that an academic world existed for them after high school. The poverty of the depression years had disappeared from most of the neighborhoods and villages of America. They had the expectations of some sort of career. They also benefited from the freedom to make that choice. Children in many parts of the world today who grow up as middle class are told by their parents what fields they can or cannot enter and what courses they should take and which, if not required, should be shunned. That American autonomy comes slowly to developing nations. But one or two generations before I was born, it was the middle-class father who decided what profession a child should have.

In this third of my generations, the expectations of careers are changing. Job security is no longer guaranteed by tradition or contract. Pensions are fast disappearing. Health insurance is uncertain. Jobs are shifting to service functions, and even skilled college-trained specialists using computers find that their jobs can be shifted to overseas graduates who will work for a fraction of the wages provided in American jobs. There is a greater burden to be creative in finding jobs more likely to last. My grandchildren are being raised in this third of my generations. Their parents both know how to cook. There is now a division of domestic labor because both parents have careers.

The Scientific Outlook Also Changes Every Generation

In 1931, the universe had recently changed from our solar system and the stars around us, including the Milky Way, to a myriad of galaxies like our Milky Way to which we belonged. We shrank even more dramatically in the cosmos than we did when Copernicus demoted us to a small planet moving in orbit around the sun. It was not known how stars produced their energy. Chemists knew a lot about small molecules, but no one knew how proteins were made from their numerous amino acids. No one knew the function of the nucleic acids in cells. Electron microscopes were not available to examine the structure of organelles in those cells or the structure of virus particles. Weather forecasting was still primitive and major storms were missed by weather bureaus. Genes could be mutated by X-rays, but no one had an idea of what was happening at a chemical level in the gene when a mutation occurred. Antibiotics did not exist, and surviving pneumonia was a matter of your body's good genes rather than the efforts of medicine. My classmates and I all experienced mumps, measles, and chicken pox. Those who were unlucky also came down with scarlet fever, polio, rheumatic fever, or a mastoid infection requiring the scraping of the cranial bone behind the ear. Some were not so lucky and died young.

By the end of my first generation, atomic energy had come into being as a threat to our lives from its military use, as an uncertain neighbor if a nuclear energy plant was to be built nearby, and as a new way to study biochemistry and treat disease. Genetics had shifted from classical to molecular. Antibiotics became diverse and abundant for eliminating the infectious diseases of my youth. Eugenics slowly died as the Depression and the Holocaust soured the public on the concept of unfit people. It was replaced by a thriving new field of human genetics. I began my conscious life listening to radio and ended my first generation watching black-and-white television. I took the train to begin graduate school in Indiana in 1953. A year later, when I got married, we flew out to Indiana with the hum of propellers roaring in my ears. I still wrote in longhand and still filled my fountain pen with ink. If I prepared a paper from my dissertation, it was on a typewriter, usually a manual one. If I needed copies, I used carbon paper between sheets of paper. My generation, after World War II ended, was very optimistic. The individual counted and could change society. Despite the Cold War, there was a feeling that freedom was spreading around the world. A middle-class or professional life was possible for all who had the talent and the drive to secure it. Unionized workers, for the first time, could live in middle-class neighborhoods.

The world view of my second generation was more guarded. The Cold War dominated political thought. Confrontation between East and West seemed inevitable. A nuclear winter was imaginable. Science shifted to multiple-authored works supported by federal money. Big science was in. It took immense machinery like cyclotrons and accelerators to study the tiniest things like atomic particles. Molecular biology spawned centrifuges, chromatography equipment, radioactive tracers, X-ray diffraction facilities, and electron microscopes. Computers became essential to analyze data. The space program extended to a landing on the moon and to explorations of our nearby planet, Mars. Telescopes became more powerful and satellite programs changed weather forecasting, spying on other countries, and identifying the features of the earth in exquisite detail. Geology shifted to plate tectonics and an understanding of mountain building, continental drift, and volcano formation and eruption. The Interstate Highway system made family travel frequent and over long distances. The truck was replacing the freight train as the best way to move goods across the country. The genetic code was worked out. Evolutionary biology added molecular biology to reconstruct the past. Macromolecules were sequenced. Molecular disease was added to the medical curriculum. Prenatal diagnosis emerged as a medical supplement, increasing the autonomy of clients to obtain and use medical information.

In my third generation, personal computers made typewriters obsolete in most offices. The Internet allowed information to flow around the world in seconds. Jet travel had forced railroads to a marginal existence for passengers. Space exploration provided detailed topographies and chemical analyses of the surfaces of the planets and their moons. Thanks to the orbiting Hubble Telescope, the universe was visible some 10–12 billion light-years away. Multiple universes were entertained, although a grand unified theory of everything in physics was still elusive. Comparative genomics and the human genome dominated molecular biology. Genes could be synthesized to order, silenced, and shifted from one species to another. Gene therapy was imagined but not yet realized. Computers had infiltrated all aspects of science. New diseases, especially AIDS, unsettled the optimism of my second generation that believed infectious diseases were a thing of the past. More women than men were going to college. The sexual revolution was ground to a halt by the appearance of AIDS. A resurgence of piety and fundamentalist-inspired world views in public affairs led to frequent attacks on evolutionary biology and the teaching of science in the public schools. The civil rights movements bogged down for those trying to extend it to homosexuals. Terrorism became the new Cold War. Religious intolerance found global expression. Science made every city and village vulnerable to harm from weapons of mass destruction. My third generation is more insecure than my first, which had seen a triumph over poverty and totalitarianism. We know in our hearts that we have been destructive to our environment, but, so far, we lack the will to bring about effective changes to show we take stewardship seriously. My third generation is a mixed history of triumphs and doubts.

What Does a Changing Human Condition Imply About Our Humanity?

I have presented the generations that I have lived. My mother-in-law, now in her 90s, presents an even stranger generation than the one I had grown up in. She shifted from a horse-and-buggy rural farm life not yet electrified to today's remarkably different world. She survived (in a blood-soaked pillow) the influenza epidemic of 1919. She knew the meaning of the term "hard times," raising her two children in the Depression. She saw the technological revolutions of the twentieth century as they occurred and the emergence of the United States as a leading world power after World War I had ended. Her first generation introduced Prohibition, jazz, the rise of labor unions, a chaotic environment of wealth through stock market speculation (more luck than merit), and the cult of hero worship through the emerging film industry. I am sure as we move back in time, one generation at a time, we would find a similar shifting of moods, novelties, reversions, and plain luck that made some generations very enjoyable and others filled with misery and uncertainty.

The human condition is almost entirely an environmentally caused state of being. It is profoundly different from our perception of human nature that we seek to make universal. Despite our efforts to have some degree of continuity, life is too diverse and the world's population (or our own country's) too immense to make such uniformity possible. If there is anything we should expect, it is change. We cannot predict what the next generation's world view will be. We have no way of anticipating new fields of science, new catastrophes, the clothing we will wear, or the music we will prefer 25 years from now. We are only good at predicting extensions from what we know. We know that at longer intervals of centuries or millennia, the changes are more dramatic and the less we have in common with civilizations or communities of preliterate people in the past.

But we do have a faith that beneath this hubbub of change, there is a rooted human being with common desires, talents, innate capacities to learn, and difficult to specify yearnings that we associate with our humanity. We recognize our desire to live, to raise a family, and to find work, love, and play in our lives. It expresses itself in different ways and it is often thwarted by circumstances we did not directly create. What is remarkable is our resilience and capacity to live with change.

Science Changes Our World Views

German scholars invented the phrase "world view" to designate how ideas and outlooks come together and are shared in a given era. A good deal of that perception of a world view was generated by the travels, findings, and writings of Alexander von Humboldt. He and his brother, also a great scholar but with an emphasis on the humanities, helped create the scholarly tradition that made German universities in the nineteenth century the most admired citadels of knowledge in the world. Humboldt was one of the last polymaths like Aristotle or Pliny the Elder who could write about the entire universe. Humboldt called his greatest work *Cosmos* to reflect this effort to tie everything together. The world view of the 1840s, when Humboldt was at his peak, was the first scientific world view. He related the forms of life he recorded as he ascended Mount Chimborazo in the Andes to the altitude and the temperature and showed that the distribution of these animals and plants was clearly limited by these factors. Darwin was inspired by Humboldt's scientific writings.

The idea that everything is connected to everything is something academics learn quickly to appreciate. Their students often have not yet learned to see the world that way. Because of their inexperience, every subject is separated by a tab not only in their notebooks, but also in their minds. World views are unifying. Their virtue is making things predictable and sensing trouble before it happens. Their drawback is that they give the illusion of permanence and they can lead to a resistance to new ideas and findings. Their self-consistency may make them seem more rational than they are.

World Views Sometimes Do Harm

What was called the Soviet empire or the countries isolated by a self-imposed iron curtain, or what President Reagan called an "evil empire," came into being after the Bolshevik revolution had deposed the Kerensky government that had just deposed the Czar and ended Russia's involvement in World War I. The Bolsheviks proclaimed a government of the proletariat—those who had been victimized for centuries by the Czars and wealthy landowners. Laborers and peasants were now the objects of government representation rather than neglect. They would be educated, housed, fed, and working, not for individual bosses, but for the state. It was a socialist vision with an eventual hope for a utopian communism in which one worked for virtue's sake and not for wages. Ideal governments are the inventions of people with good intentions who minimize the diversity of the people who would live in such states. For Lenin and other architects of the Bolshevik revolution, it was a planned society. Science would play a major role in lifting the USSR out of its ancient past and into the modern world. Factories would be built to catapult Russia into the twentieth century as an industrial power. Dams would be built to prevent floods and irrigate farmland. Farms would be collectivized and mechanized, doing away with practices closer to medieval times than to the twentieth century. The state would decide what it needed through its hierarchical structure leading upward to one central figure, Lenin himself, or his successor Stalin. The difficulty with such a system where all the parts fit together on flowcharts and diagrams is that the people are not plug-ins to some mental pegboard. They have ideas of their own, different aspirations, different personalities, and different talents. When the state or its subsidiaries take over, that freedom to explore, to learn from mistakes, to change course in one's career, or to be creative can be stifled or rendered as criminal or antisocial behavior.

The world view of the "thousand year Reich" was equally flawed. Hitler created a national socialist state in which his monomania saw a Nazi world of one people, one state, and one leader. It was unashamedly authoritarian, in contrast to the hypocrisy of Soviet communism that pretended to be a democracy. It also claimed to be the first state based on biological principles. What a perversion those alleged principles were with a ranking of people according to race, with a subspecies designation of those most reviled by Hitler and his party theorists, and with scientists of good standing used to promote programs of compulsory sterilization and euthanasia of those designated as "the unfit." Yet, to many a Nazi who joined willingly and enthusiastically in the late 1920s and 1930s, the entire system was harmonious. It provided jobs during the depression years. It provided generous paid maternity leaves for women who worked. It provided free health care for children. It provided paid vacations to spas for laboring families. It created the affordable car, the Volkswagen, and the highway system to connect working-class Germans with their families. It repudiated the Versailles treaty and it restored Germany to its military glory. Everything was connected. But those who rejoiced at the new vigor of Germany were soon awakened to a different reality. To make it work, there had to be a Gestapo to keep an eye on dissidents. To make it work, there had to be a closed government rather than an open one, and so a free press disappeared. To make it work, there had to be a war even more vicious and with greater carnage than in World War I. It would mean a decimation of the manhood of Germany as their boys were taken from their families and shifted to the Russian front to be killed in the millions.

History is littered with failed world views, most of them associated with expansionist dreams of empire. Dante's view of a single Christendom extending to all corners of the world was such a scheme. Despite the evidence of warfare among different states in the emerging Europe of his day, he naïvely believed that under a single Christian world, such conflicts would cease because the Pope would be the titular head of the world. One-world utopian thinking has been a recurrent theme, mostly of philosophers. Despite initial optimism, world federations such as the League of Nations or the United Nations have not yet won the support of governments who do not wish to surrender part of their sovereignty to democratize international decision-making. Some are harmful because of their hidden agendas of controlling diversity of thought and cultures.

Other world views are not imposed by empire builders or idealists who manage to bring about their visions. They emerge because of changing social institutions and cultures. The world view of an American living in 1880 was quite different from one living in 1980. In 1880, that person would almost certainly be a white Anglo-Saxon Protestant male, a descendant of ancestors who predated the American Revolution, with national rather than international outlooks. In 1880, that person would see a future in developing the western part of America, displacing Native Americans who were not already chased across the Mississippi River into ever more isolated reservations. In 1980, that person could be a male or a female, Protestant or Catholic, with ancestry more likely to have come over in the previous 80 years. That person would have an international outlook (we were still in the Cold War), would worry about nuclear war and annihilation, and would feel awkward about the gains won by blacks and women but would be open to their presence in politics and the professions.

How Science Changes World Views

Science changes our world views in several ways. The germ theory of the 1880s led to a sanitary movement in the industrial nations of the world. This led to a dramatic drop in infant mortality and a mushrooming population. The generations facing large families that were unplanned sought a way out and embraced planned parenthood and the birth control movement. This reduced the family size back to what it was in the old days when death from infectious diseases of children was part of the reality of life. I doubt if either Louis Pasteur or Robert Koch had ever considered that applications of their germ theory of infectious diseases would lead to a population explosion. Thus, some world views emerge as unintended consequences of scientific findings.

Science can also change world views by discoveries that are in conflict with contemporary beliefs. The work of Copernicus and Galileo overthrew a central location in people's minds of where earth ranked in the universe. Putting it third among the planets around the sun was a psychological shock, but it also was considered heretical by both the Pope and Luther. Religions had not yet come to accept science when science conflicted with religious traditions. It took two more centuries for those older views of a central huge earth to die out. Because so little of our knowledge of the universe was a consequence of scientific effort before the 1500s, the number of conflicts was limited to a world based on the five senses. Microscopy did not conflict with religious world views. The revelation of more stars and planets as telescopes increased in power did not cause consternation for religion. By the 1920s and 1930s, when an expanding universe consisting of huge numbers of galaxies as big as our Milky Way were observed by Hubble and other astronomers, the process of reducing the earth to a mote within a mote in the universe was no longer shocking.

Conflicts did emerge over findings in biology. It was upsetting when compounds found in living things could be synthesized by organic chemists. It was shocking when embryologists showed that they could produce artificial twins and what that would imply for human cloning. It was shocking when chimeras were found among humans with ambiguous sexual anatomy and XX and XY cells suggesting that what should have been two people, brother and sister twins, were one individual. How such individuals are to be interpreted legally and theologically is still much disputed. It was shocking when the technologies of prenatal diagnosis and in vitro fertilization became part of standard medical practice. It was shocking when chemical, hormonal, and mechanical devices could be used safely to prevent pregnancies from occurring.

Scientists have synthesized viruses from off-the-shelf chemicals. They have introduced genes from one phylum into another phylum. They have worked out the sequence of nucleotides in our entire genome. They have provided evidence for evolution by natural selection for more than one and a half centuries. These are like bombshells during a siege. These discoveries and developments collectively created a materialist view of life free of entelechies, mnemes, homunculi, vitalistic essences, holistic structures incapable of analysis by science, and other supernatural agencies that allegedly generated life in the past. For those who see these immaterial essences as flowing from God's finger in Michelangelo's representation of Adam's creation, these are unsettling findings.

Coping With Changing World Views

We have limited capacities to predict the future, but we have few limits on extending what we know into the future. The world has many countries and many cultures so there are coexisting as well as competitive world views from a global perspective. The perspective of the Islamic world, although diverse when carefully examined, does share an expansionist outlook. Islam and the state are more intimately connected than Christianity and the state are connected today. To westerners, Islam is similar to Christian attitudes during the era of the Crusades and the voyages of exploration and conquest that attempted to Christianize those in Africa, Asia, and the New World. Today, such expansionist views of Christianity are rare or nonexistent. Most European states are secular. Governments are considered independent of religion even when the country's constitution endorses a national religion. This is not true of many of the Islamic states where there is a close cooperation, if not unity, between the goals of the state and the goals of its leading religious leaders. How this conflict between a secular outlook in the industrial nations and a theocratic outlook in many of the nonindustrial nations will play out is not predictable. Often, we have to experience the future rather than recognize what it will be.

Scientists dread any conflict with religion because they feel that it is not their intent to be at war with religion. Their intention is to be objective about how the world works. If there are contradictions against popular or religious belief, that may be unfortunate, but scientists feel an obligation to their fields and not to the prevailing and sometimes erroneous views of faith-based beliefs. Although it may take centuries for religions to accommodate the findings of science, in the long run, they do. No major scientific finding has been successfully suppressed or abandoned because it contradicts the theology of specific religions.

What type of world view might emerge in this third millennium that will be science-dominated? At the scale of the very large, we may have more clarity about the existence of more than one type of universe. Multiuniverse (or multiverse) proponents believe that they are possible because mathematical modeling permits their existence and that they would have physical properties somewhat different from those that exist in our own universe. With or without multiuniverses, the concept of our own universe is still daunting in its immensity. One of the difficulties of cosmology is the lack of data to distinguish among contending models. As the flood of data pours in from future telescopes set up on the moon or in space stations, it will narrow the number of contending models of our universe. For most of humanity, there would be little contradiction to their place in the universe as these contending models are pared down. At the scale of the very small, our outlook about the composition of atoms and their particles may be resolved if tests of string theory support it or eliminate it from contention. Because we humans do not sense or concern ourselves at this incredibly minute level of existence, it is unlikely that our place in the universe will be threatened or profoundly changed.

The far more important impacts of science will be at the level that touches our lives. In the life sciences, interests in both health and the natural life cycle we experience will be filled with new surprises as scientists learn how a fertilized egg unfolds, cell division by cell division to sort out its molecular changes and acquisition of new functions. Every organ system will someday be interpreted at a molecular level, and the possibility of making our own organ replacements will apply to vital organs with the exception of our entire brain. We may augment or replace damaged parts of our brains but we cannot conceive of a way to restore lost memories and skills that were present in billions of neurons that were destroyed by disease. I am doubtful if science will ever find a way of arresting the aging process or arresting the production of spontaneous mutations in our germ line or in our somatic tissues. Staying 29 years old for a millennium or more may appeal to the imagination of wishful thinkers, but any reflections on the consequences of such an option will reveal its impossibility or moral injustices. It would force humanity to forego having children because if most of the living elected not to age or die, there would be no resources on earth sufficient to maintain such a population of self-centered people for all the things that would fill their centuries with activities that were not tiresome repetitions of what they experienced in the past. It would be a Midas touch of life.

Much more realistic will be the advances in diagnosis and treatment of conditions that prematurely shorten our lives. Our mean life expectancy may increase by another 10 years, but it is difficult to imagine healthy vigorous people in their 90s and 100s when they will soon die from the aging process. Most people in those advanced years find they need assisted living and have not been employed for a generation. No doubt there will be more studies in gerontology on the activities such a significant percentage of the world population can do. This includes opportunities for volunteer work, which could be important in reducing the anticipated expenses of an aged retired population no longer generating the money for its needs.

That emerging world view will see science as essential to solving complex problems. It will include an ethic of stewardship not only for the environment, but also for our own bodies. It will stress the importance of opening potentials we have, rather than limiting them through neglect. Science tends to be optimistic about the uses of its knowledge. It will also be a more moral world because the idea of fairness, of the Golden Rule or its Kantian reason-based equivalent, is more attractive in secular governments than faith-based specific religious values that are usually a subset of the contending values found among all religions.

Recommended Reading

A very comprehensive view of how nineteenth-century thought formed a world view can be found in John Theodore Merz's *A history of European thought in the nineteenth century* (1903. W. Blackwood and Sons, Edinburgh). His book is a trove of attitudinal changes in science and society.

Numerous books abound on failed world views. William Shirer's *The rise and fall of the Third Reich* (1960. Simon and Schuster, New York) is representative of several other failed world views, such as the Communist dreams of the now defunct USSR. Not all collapse from their own ideological demands. Some cannot compete with new ways of living.

CHAPTER 17

Rethinking Science Teaching

I HAVE ARGUED THAT SCIENCE WILL DOMINATE CULTURE in the third millennium. Dealing with the problems of neglect, the problems of applying new knowledge, and the problems of technology of mass destruction in wars, terrorism, and civil insurgencies require effective citizenship and informed legislators. How should one teach the science we need to know to be effective citizens? Our present methods of teaching are based on a twentieth-century model of education that isolates the science from the things to which it is applied. Scientists are used to abstract thinking, and it is easy to forget that children and teenagers are not very good at abstract reasoning. They need to be weaned from concrete to abstract approaches rather than plunged directly into a "sink-or-swim" model that is characteristic of many science courses. A second distinction involves college-level science courses for those who intend to become scientists versus courses for those who are only taking a science course as a way to fulfill a requirement for their breadth of knowledge component of their undergraduate education. In many smaller colleges, there is only one course, the majors course, because the college does not have the funds to hire additional faculty to teach nonmajors courses. There is virtually no interdisciplinary science for the citizen course that blends biology, chemistry, physics, astronomy, and geology into a 1-year course. Yet, many colleges offer such interdisciplinary humanities courses that cover western civilization or world civilizations from a philosophic, historical, literary, artistic, political, and comparative religious perspective.

There are many reasons why teaching for effective citizenship is difficult. We are trained to be specialists and not generalists. Few scientists read so widely and have sufficient understanding of fields outside their own specialty that they would want to teach such a course. Most colleges that try these interdisciplinary approaches use team-taught courses where the segments are taught by specialists. The hope of the organizers of these courses is that somehow students will see the connections across the disciplines. In some programs, one faculty member in the team becomes a "master learner" who attends all of the lectures and helps the students make those associations. Some schools do this at the entry level in the first year. Others use the senior year for "capstone" seminars to bring what the student has learned over the years to the issues that require interdisciplinary approaches for solution. Newly designed courses do not have textbooks for them and collections of books or articles are used in their stead.

Learning Science to Become an Informed Citizen

I have spent most of my academic life teaching nonscience majors. I made the shift about 1964 when I interviewed many students as UCLA's premedical advisor. I was impressed by their idealism; some of them were the first returnees from the newly established Peace Corps. One was a theater arts major who had been sent to the Philippines to teach English literature. After a few weeks on the job, he told his supervisor that two of his students were missing. He was told that they had died. He was stunned. The students had died of infectious diseases. "How can I teach English if my students are dying?" he asked his supervisor. His supervisor transferred him to a field station that served some 300,000 people in a rural area. He was given texts of parasitology to read and was taught how to use a microscope. He came back desiring to take the courses he needed to apply to medical school so he could return and make a difference.

I was moved by a sign taped to the window in the student union, "Why take a history course this summer? Be history! Join the voter registration drive in Mississippi." I wondered why issues like race were discussed without some knowledge of the genetic differences that lead to changes in skin color among populations. I wondered why wars were fought and if aggression was learned or genetically on tap from our past animal ancestry. I wondered what happens in a psychotic's brain that makes him kill our president or other national leaders. I wondered how we could enter a debate over radioactive fallout when the science behind those issues was reduced to slogans that were misleading. I wondered if there was a population bomb about to go off or if this was a recurrent Malthusian pessimism. I wondered about the effects of contaminating chemicals in our water supplies, food, and the air we breathe. Was the construction of a nuclear reactor near a large city a wise decision? How does one evaluate these? Did what I teach inform citizens to sort out conflicting claims? How should the citizen be educated about science?

I realized that the way nonscience students learn science is flawed. They get what is often called a "watered-down" majors course. Making a course less demanding is not the best way to teach. I designed a nonmajors course that I called "Biology: A Humanities Approach." I wanted students to know the following five major ideas about biology: (1) Life is composed of cells, (2) life is an outcome of genes, (3) organisms have a life cycle, (4) all living things evolve, and (5) there is a molecular basis to life. I then asked what examples from the news media could I introduce to show how one or more of these five concepts was needed to understand the issue. For radiation from fallout and other sources, it was knowledge of genes and chromosomes and their relation to cell division. I could describe mitosis as it happens in normal dividing cells and then describe it for a cell whose chromosome has been broken by ionizing radiation. Such cells enter what is called a breakage-fusion-bridge cycle and kill the cell. If a lot of cells are exposed to radiation at some intensity as in Hiroshima and Nagasaki, the tissues of our adult bodies that have dividing cells such as skin, gut, bone marrow, and the lining of our vascular system are the most vulnerable to dying of these abnormal cell divisions. This produces the cluster of symptoms called radiation sickness. When taught in this way, mitosis is placed in a context of the student's awareness and suddenly they understand why radiation protection is needed during times when heavy doses of radiation are present.

When discussing the life cycle, I would use the first 55 days of pregnancy called organogenesis to tell not only how an embryo is formed from a fertilized egg, but also what happens to the embryo when it is exposed to thalidomide, leading to malformations that are quite severe. Students then learn that there are agents called teratogens and young women can protect themselves by memorizing the phrase—Has this product been tested for teratogenicity?—whenever they are given a prescription. The most vulnerable stage of pregnancy is when the woman does not know she is pregnant or she doesn't look pregnant, and a health care provider might not think of asking about the possibility of being pregnant.

In teaching this course for more than 35 years, the five major concepts did not change, but the issues of the day constantly shifted. This shows that creating informed citizens is less about talking about what side to take on the controversial issues than about the science needed to understand why they are controversial. I did not preach about who is right or wrong on a controversial issue. My job was to give the students the science in the context of the debate so that they could understand it in a more informed way. It is more about using reason, facts, and an understanding of how things work than about being politically left or right. The mistake many teachers make is that if these issues are analyzed the way I describe, they think they are obliged to tell students what their outlook should be. Americans are too diverse for such a slanting of knowledge for political purposes. If you show how science is used by one group, such as Edward Teller in the radiation controversy, you see he argues from the perspective of the individual risk to damage from extremely low doses. Linus Pauling uses the same data, but he does it from the perspective of the total inferred victims from the entire world's population. Getting students to see how science is used in these controversies is what I believe makes good citizens.

The Media Should Play a Greater Role in Covering Science

We also cannot rely on teaching alone to do this job. If we look at a major newspaper such as *The New York Times*, its opinion page is filled with commentaries on politics, economics, racial issues, popular culture interests, and occasional topics of the day. It is rare for science commentary to be seen in those pages (about one article every 2 or 3 weeks). But *The New York Times* does set aside a section on science each Tuesday, and it is very good in conveying the week's news of science gleaned from *Science, Nature,* and other periodicals, or from national meetings of science specialty groups. Compare this to the coverage each day on films, books, music, art shows, restaurants, and the things that consume most of our interests—business, real estate, sports, food, and fashion. It would be an error to make the schools the only source for science knowledge. Just as these daily interests are spread across the week and written for the public, rather than fellow specialists, we need more science tucked into articles about things that matter. It is not just health and the environment or the military applications of scientific knowledge that deserve attention.

Science probes how we think, how we perceive the outside world, how we lived millennia or tens of millennia ago, and how our view of life, the material world, and our values are being challenged by science. If we were to tabulate what is devoted to the pages of our newspapers and magazines or to what is available to see on our television sets, we would find that the portion devoted to the science in our lives is vastly under-represented. There are many reasons for this. Science, if presented as isolated from human activities and interests, will not be read or watched by those who hate science or fear it. It will turn off most readers or viewers if it is boring or presented like encyclopedia articles. Journalists can be very skilled in presenting the things that interest readers. Not many journalists, however, have enough science background to assess the quality of science they report.

Dealing with the Conflicts of Science and Religion

The controversial issues that involve environmentalism and health are far easier to teach and provide the science involved in them and how they are used and occasionally misused through ignorance, failure to test adequately, or use of inadequate experimentation. What is very difficult to do is to present the world view of science when it deals with issues that clash with the world view of religions rooted in a past belief about the way life works and its history. Those who believe humans were placed as humans on earth and did not evolve are not interested in hearing the evidence for natural selection, the fossil record, comparative anatomy, comparative genomics, or any evidence that science offers in attempting to construct a history of life on earth. Natural history does not exist in their world view. *Genesis* exists, and it is seen not as a religious book, but as an historical document of how the universe came into being, and whatever is present in that text is seen as irrefutable because it was dictated by God to Moses. When introducing this in my biology course for nonmajors, I stated my position as clearly as I could. I told the class that I was a scientist and as a scientist I had an obligation to teach what I learned and what I believe to be representative of good science. One of those aspects involves the evolution of life on earth. I told them that they were free to reject it if their faith-based beliefs were contradicted, but it was my job as a scientist neither to leave it out nor to distort it so it would not seem to contradict their beliefs. I told them no matter how much they rejected evolution, they should at least know what they are rejecting and not some straw-man model of evolution they learned in Sunday school.

I also emphasized, when I introduced the concept of birth defects and how they occur, that the responses to such pregnancies varied. Some do not want to undergo prenatal diagnosis because of their religious beliefs which associates such procedures with elective abortions. I told them that was fine. That was their choice based on their values. But I told them that this is a democracy with many religions. Many of them considered prenatal diagnosis with elective abortion to be an acceptable procedure if done with an examined conscience. I told them that all couples, whatever their religious beliefs, do a lot of reflecting about such personal crises. They may choose not to have more children. They may choose prenatal diagnosis. They may choose to adopt instead of passing on a hereditary defect. They may choose a sperm or egg donor if the condition is known to come from only one of the parents. They may feel that it is not theirs to choose but God's will or fate and they will take their chances and rely on prayer. All of these are likely to happen in a democracy. It ceases to be a democracy when one group imposes a ban on what others can do. Theocracies and pluralistic democracies are not very compatible.

One of the major difficulties that scientists face when expanding their outreach to a wider public is the way science is taught in K–12 classrooms. Parents are aware that young children are very vulnerable to accepting whatever they learn in school as true. They are not taught to doubt, to question, to weigh evidence. It is not easy with students whose brains are still forming and who lack the developmental maturity of their brains to handle abstract ideas and controversies. Thus, parents prefer no teaching of controversies at all for fear that their children will take positions contrary to their parents' political or religious beliefs. Schools are very sensitive to such pressures from voters who can elect school board members with views hostile to science. They can also mobilize the vote to reject school budgets, making it difficult for schools to function. In a curious way, parents who have such strong feelings do not realize they are cheating students of becoming good citizens who can assess what is reason-based and what is faith-based, what uses a political slant and what constitutes an actual scientific finding. Whatever will be done in reforming science education will come about gradually because of this resistance that can last several generations unless a crisis of international scope, like the Sputnik satellite of 1957 or perhaps the current climate change issue, suddenly galvanizes school districts, Congress, and science advocacy groups to urge action in such a moment of turmoil.

That likely reaction by a determined minority governed by faith-based beliefs is a major reason why I feel that both our educational programs and our mass media coverage need to work together to bring about the science literacy of the third millennium. Scientists also have to educate themselves about this need. Without an informed electorate, they are at risk of seeing bad laws enacted, serious problems neglected, and funding for basic science gutted by those who feel threatened by science. Scientists are also citizens who vote and have opinions using values that are faith-based even if they are secular ones. They have to reflect on ways to teach science without making the mistakes of the early twentieth century. When the government uses science to endorse its viewpoints, Holocausts can occur on a large scale or compulsory sterilization laws to eliminate alleged degenerates from breeding can be enacted on a more limited scale. When science invites the government to take sides on a debate and choose between two contending scientific claims, as in the notorious Lysenko controversy of 1935–1965, an entire generation may be deprived of a legitimate science, as happened when the Communist Party endorsed Lysenko's Michurinism to replace classical genetics, which Lysenkoists regarded as bourgeois, fascist, and divorced from socialist reality.

Living with complexity when our minds yearn for simplicity is not easy. Teaching that complexity inherent in controversies is also filled with risks. Teachers who hope to share their enthusiasm for the rational way science can be used to tease apart the complex and assist us in understanding what is going on have to plan their lectures carefully to make sure that they do not damage the reputation of science (or themselves) by going beyond those reason-based arguments. Yet, in facing that choice, I chose those risks as part of the satisfaction of making my students aware of how science gave them the very outcome intended in a liberal arts education. It made them use reason-based thinking and made them recognize that although science had no monopoly on such an approach, it could not exist without it.

Recommended Reading

This is a field where much of the information is transmitted through conferences and workshops, rather than books. For about 17 years, the Lilly Endowment held workshops on the liberal arts at Colorado College. During those 2 weeks, faculty teams from about 20 colleges each year would share ideas and seek advice on innovative programs. I knew of only one college, Millsap College, in Jackson, Mississippi, that tried to introduce an integrated general science course similar to that of a Columbia University "Contemporary Civilization of the West" course. Many schools do introduce science and society courses through senior capstone courses or through programs called Federated Learning Communities where a master learner faculty member attempts to coordinate cognate faculty around a common theme such as "World hunger" or "Science, ethics, and the liberal arts."

CHAPTER 18

A Human Outlook for the Third Millennium

THE HUMAN CONDITION IS OURS TO SHAPE. Whatever may be said about human nature, whether it describes us sourly as steeped in original sin, "nasty and brutish," or driven by evolutionary programs that served our world for 90% of our existence as the genus *Homo,* or whether we flatter ourselves as being "a little lower than the angels," our self-perception limits us more often than it opens us to the possibility of being in charge, of having the capacity to change for the better. Just consider how different we are in self-perception than our ancestors were a few centuries ago. How could we have accepted child labor or slavery unless we took a dim view of the human nature of those who were abused? How could we have tolerated the denial of education and professional occupation to women unless we had a very limited idea of how talents were distributed by our alleged sexual natures? How could we live for centuries with the vast majority of humanity deprived of an education or a voice in their own governance? Do not those views reflect false perceptions of human nature? Do we not divide humanity into privileged groups and losers and rationalize all of this in our minds by religious sanction, living out of the sins of ancestors, or being cursed as a class of people for seeing Noah drunk and naked? Did not our pastors' or priests' sermons justify the privileged to exploit others and to accept the base nature of most of humanity or the harsh judgment of God?

We live our lives in three tenses: present, past, and future. The present occupies our careers and family life. The past gives us a connection to our communities, ancestry, and national identity. The future gives us those goals and ideals that motivate us as we move along the trajectory of our present human life cycle of some four score years and some. We can classify time in another way. We live our lives in generational times (going back to grandparents and looking ahead to grandchildren). We may have been too young to remember great-grandparents if we were lucky enough to have been born while they were still alive. We are likely to be too old to appreciate our great-grandchildren, especially if we are in our frail 80s or 90s when they are born.

We also live in historical time. Mine spans the years of the great Depression to the era of unexpected terrorism. We shape our lives around world events and national events that can powerfully alter our lives. Least familiar to us, because of our profound isolation from the science that surrounds us, is our sense of evolutionary time. It connects us to our origins and to the diversity of life that exists on earth and an even greater diversity that has, at best, left traces of its former extent in the fossil record. It also vastly increases our awareness of time, the impermanence of things, and the vulnerability of life.

The evolutionary sense of time is rarely invoked in Congress and the White House, and in all likelihood, it is muted in the Supreme Court. Our governments live in generational time, not evolutionary time. Without that sense of evolutionary time, concepts such as global warming, the hazards of mutations from nuclear war, the accidental or deliberate introduction of animals and plants not native to a continent or an island, or the consequences of cutting down forests without replacing them are not likely to be taken seriously. The bad outcomes are more likely to occur long after a general, congressional committee head, cabinet member, judge, or corporation board member has died and been forgotten.

Our sense of size is also distorted because of our size and the way our sense organs have evolved to live in a world where predators have to be sufficiently large to be seen. We did not evolve eyes to see germs. We rely instead on our immune systems. But both our immune systems and the germs that make us sick or kill us also evolve. We saw evolution in action when a new species of virus, HIV, arose about 30 or 40 years ago in Africa, finding a new host in humans from a simian ancestor virus. AIDS has entered every continent and continues to kill millions of people worldwide, but because we have a limited knowledge of biology and evolution, we look for moral solutions to medical problems. "Just say no" does not work as well as condoms. Bad science (or self-deception) is used to smear the far greater effectiveness of using condoms as a preventive of transmitting the virus than "just say no." When insisting on an ideal of universal virtue (through abstinence) to the reality that semiliterate and ignorant youth will experiment with sex as they have in all generations past is an act of murdering those youths for the crime of fornication. Is killing others in wars, insurrections, and other turmoil a lesser evil than allowing young people to die for having sex outside of monogamous marriage? Before there was an AIDS pandemic, were young people more virtuous than they are today?

Because we cannot see our cells, chromosomes, and genes, we are unaware of the damage done to individual genes, chromosomes, or cells. When genes are altered, their likelihood of having harmful effects on development or metabolism is far greater than of benefiting the child who is conceived from such a new mutation. Our knowledge of genetics can make us more concerned about effective testing of what enters our mouths, lungs, and skins. A balance between risk and cost can be worked out in society. Without that knowledge, manufacturers just see added costs and everything is perceived through a filter of economics.

We can understand why our sense of size was so limited until the sixteenth century, when telescopes were introduced, and a century later, the first microscopes were being used. They were crude by today's standards, but the first findings revealed the world of the very small and the world of the very large and far away. Without science and optics to give us instruments to see these worlds, we would have remained with the illusion that the earth is the largest object in the universe and nothing was smaller than a mustard seed. Our sense of size changed even when we were vaguely aware of the solar system and the existence of an industrial revolution taking place in cities far away. I was reminded of that when entering the doors of a home that is now a museum in Setauket. The Thompson House was built about 1700 or shortly before that and it has been restored. Going from room to room, I had to lower my head. I am 5 feet 11 inches tall and not many people were of that height in the early 1700s. I was equally surprised at the size of adult bodies when I looked at the suits of armor in the Metropolitan Museum of Art. They are of a size that we would expect to fit today's 13- or 14-year-old boys. Those changes have occurred in historical time, not evolutionary time, so the shift in our body size as a result of the germ theory and the immense improvements of mechanized farming and nutrition are dramatic compared to the gradual increase over tens or hundreds of millennia in size that took place during the transition from the earliest members of walking primates, *Australopithecines* and early *Homo*.

It was not until the twentieth century that our size shifted to the molecular level, and we could visualize the structure of our proteins and our DNA. I have not framed a photo of a segment of my DNA, although I do know some colleagues who have done so. My wife was given a present by her co-workers of two framed photographs of her 46 chromosomes and my 46 chromosomes as they appear spread out but prior to being cut out and aligned in size place. We have displayed this family photo under a lamp in our living room for many years, and it is a reminder of how we would look if humanity had the capacity to see itself at that microscopic level. It is a reminder that trillions of such cells are in each of our bodies and that just as we have a stewardship over the care of our bodies at the familiar level of everyday living, we also have to have a stewardship to protect those chromosomes from agents that break them or mutate them. Without knowledge of science, that stewardship becomes doubtful.

We are fortunate that the world of larger things has been brought home by NASA and other national space programs. Sending humans to the moon required a lot of engineering skills and scientific understanding of living in a cramped environment for the 2 weeks or so of those trips. It takes years to launch a mission to Mars and other planets. Unless spaceships can be accelerated to speeds several orders of magnitude faster than they are now, human travel to the farther planets such as Jupiter and Saturn and a return to Earth is not likely to take place. Astronauts would be spending decades just traveling each way. It is even more remote that we will visit planets of our nearest stars until a technology of near speed of light travel becomes possible. Realizing science fiction fantasies requires a technology that does not yet exist.

As enormous as the size becomes when we think about traveling about our solar system and getting close-up pictures of planetary surfaces and their moons, we are humbled by the size of our galaxy, the distances between galaxies, and the stupendous number of galaxies in our universe. Imagining that vast amount of matter and realizing that virtually all of those galaxies contain as many stars as our own Milky Way galaxy makes it difficult to believe that our little earth in this sea of matter is the only place where intelligent life has evolved. Think for a moment about the contrast between a human looking at the world in 1400 and seeing the earth as immensely huge compared to anything else in the visible skies. Then think of a dot virtually on the edge of disappearing from view in Carl Sagan's image of our planet as seen from a space vehicle beyond the planets but still within our solar system and far away from our nearest neighboring star. Then reflect that what he called "the pale blue dot" is not even seen when our sun is just lost in a myriad of other stars if we could look at our galaxy a few tens of thousands of light-years from where we are. And then reflect that if our Milky Way galaxy were to be seen one billion or more light-years away on another galaxy, it would be invisible without a superb astronomical telescope and it would be just one of many miniscule spinning whirligigs in space. What is thrilling of this image of ourselves in this universe is that science gave us the capacity to understand it and find out where we are in our galaxy and what our immediate and farther neighboring galaxies look like.

Our sense of size also evolves. The log cabin home my wife's great-grandmother lived in as a girl in Fulton County, Indiana, is still around and now a museum display in their Historical Society. It is not very large and reminds us how our sense of what size we should expect our living quarters to be has changed in a little over a century. Every time I go to New York City and stay over in a Manhattan apartment, I am reminded how much smaller those living quarters are compared to the space of homes in the suburbs. Community and personal space change also with the era and place in which we live. As a young adult going to college at New York University, I often ate my dinner in an Automat, a cafeteria where several nickels or quarters could deliver a beef pie, a cake, or hot dogs and beans. I would take my tray of food and then sit at a table, empty if I were lucky but soon to be visited by a stranger. During the crowded eating hours, there would be four strangers at one table, eating in silence, respecting the privacy of each other. People were not rude. They realized that they would never see each other again and so it was not necessary to engage in small talk for the 10 or 15 minutes that their four personal spaces came together at one table.

In addition to challenging our sense of time and size, science has challenged our sense of what we familiarly call the material world around us and that composes us. We are mostly unaware of how molecules combine or how they are taken apart in our cells. We have a vague idea that food is recycled, but before the 1850s and the first forays of physiology into our metabolism, we had no idea what was going on. Food came in one end and liquid and semisolid waste came out the other end. Learning that we break up foods into their smaller molecules and recycle them took a lot of experimentation. Learning that the process involves both the use of energy to make more complex molecules and the production of energy by oxidizing smaller circulating molecules through our mitochondria was a twentieth-century accomplishment. I was forcefully made aware of that when my father-in-law died in 1968. As I approached his open casket, I placed my hand on his folded journeyman's hands. They were cold, at room temperature, or slightly chilled by the refrigeration where he had been stored. My hands had the hidden fire of life churning out ATP and other energy-rich molecules from my mitochondria. His mitochondria were silent, shut off, no new molecules being taken apart or put together by his ATP. Death had a molecular presence at that moment as our hands touched. Less than 50 years earlier, death would have been limited to an organ's failure—a stilled unbeating heart, lungs that no longer shoved air in or out, a brain unresponsive to sound, touch, or other stimulation. Experiencing death at this molecular level enriched my appreciation of what life is and what distinguishes meat from living flesh.

The world of matter outside our bodies has also changed profoundly throughout the twentieth century as physicists described atoms, radioactivity, atomic particles with charges, uncharged atomic particles, and the use of neutrons released in atomic decay to produce atomic energy or atomic weapons of mass destruction. Just as the very large and the very far away give us distances that stun our imaginations in the astronomer's world, the world of atomic particles, forces that hold atoms together, and ultimate theoretical strings that may have been the first precursor of matter of the universe also provide a new way to see ourselves through the discoveries of science. The lessons for those who take seriously their stewardship of life and the planet we live on are different for those whose sense of science is shallow and for whom weapons of mass destruction are perceived as implements for ideological fanaticism or questionable ethics at best. Science becomes abused when it is separated from values that foster our survival, that recognize the right to live of those who disagree with us in religion, politics, or world views.

It becomes abused when we elevate profits, jobs, a lobbyist's quid pro quo, or convenience and habit over the health, aesthetic pleasure of living, or quality of environment that innocent people may have to pay for those short-term gains.

Being fully human requires the union of values and a science-based awareness of who we are. Human nature is not just words and ideas debated back and forth by theologians and philosophers who lived centuries or millennia ago. Human nature is the realization that humans have evolved a self-awareness, a use of reason to survive, an imagination that gives us values allowing us to live together, an empathy to understand the triumphs and tragedies others experience, and the potential to be creative. We maintain our dreams and ideals while we raise our families and invest hopes in our future as an ever-vulnerable species, stumbling over our errors, ignorance, and prejudices, but enjoying our capability to visit the moon and neighboring planets, describe the double helix of DNA, produce theories of relativity and the quantum atom, and compose Beethoven's *Ninth Symphony*, Dostoevsky's *Brothers Karamazov*, Van Gogh's *Starry Night*, Michelangelo's *David*, and Plato's *Apology*.

Recommended Reading

Carl Sagan's two most provocative books I felt were *The cosmic connection: An extraterrestrial perspective* (1973. Anchor Press, Garden City, New York) (where he makes us aware that we are "star children" born of the elements blown out from dying stars), and *The pale blue dot: A vision of the human future in space* (1994. Random House, New York), where Sagan makes us see ourselves from one of our farthermost rockets at the edge of the solar system.

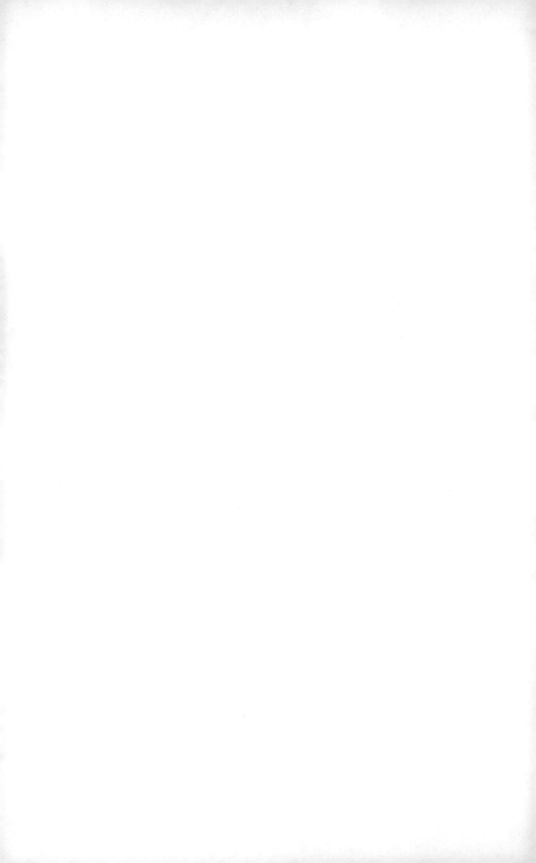

Index

evidence for claims, 121–123
  fallacy, 119–121, 126
blank slate fallacy, 107–108
community formation, 127–131
definition, 173
evolutionary psychology, 115–119
versus human condition, 2–3
religious versus secular view,
  113–115
Humanities. *See* Arts and humanities
Huntington disease, 69

I

Immigration, Americans, 3–4
Intelligence
  assessment difficulties, 123–126
  genetic factors, 110–111
Intelligent design, 56

K

Kant, Immanual, 141–142
Kinsey, Alfred, 131
Kohlberg, Lawrence, 139

L

Lamarck, Jean Baptiste, 42
Lawrence, D.H., 136
Lenin, Vladimir, 152
Lewis, Edward B., 85
Linnaeus, Carl, 43
LSD, 101
Lysenko, Trofim, 31 32
Lysosome, 50

M

Mangold, Hilde, 44
Marlowe, Christopher, 135
Material world, denial and harm, 28–30
Melanin, 66–67
Mendel, Gregor, 45, 66–68, 70
Merleau-Ponty, Maurice, 99
Mitochondria, 50
Mitochondrial DNA, 59–60
Mitosis, discovery, 48
Molecular genetics
  evolutionary history studies, 80–82

gene replacement therapy, 78–79
historical perspective, 75–78
prenatal diagnosis, 78
Moral values
  community binding, 139–144
  reason-based moral codes, 141–144
  Ten Commandments, 140–141
  utilitarian ethics, 143
Muller, Hermann, 57, 65
Mullerian duct, 90

N

Nationalism, 33
Necrogenetics, 81
Neurobiology
  brain
    empirical findings of function,
      100–101
    mind theory, 101–103
  historical perspective, 97–99
  synapse, 99–100
Newton, Isaac, 19
NMR. *See* Nuclear magnetic resonance
Nuclear magnetic resonance
  (NMR), 98

O

Opsins, 80–81
Origin of Species, 58
Original sin, 113–114

P

Paley, William, 56
Paracelsus, 135
Parthenogenesis, 84
Pauling, Linus, 162
Penfield, Wilder, 100
Pepys, Samuel, 97
PET. *See* Positron emission
  tomography
Positron emission tomography (PET), 98
Preformation, 83–84
Prenatal diagnosis, 78, 164
Pseudogene, 80
Pseudohermaphrodite, 92–93
Psychology, 98